❖ REMOVING THE ROADBLOCKS ❖
Group Psychotherapy with Substance Abusers and Family Members

The Guilford Substance Abuse Series

EDITORS

HOWARD T. BLANE, Ph.D.
Research Institute on Alcoholism, Buffalo

THOMAS R. KOSTEN, M.D.
Yale University School of Medicine, New Haven

❖ REMOVING THE ❖ ROADBLOCKS

Group Psycotherapy with
Substance Abusers and
Family Members

MARSHA VANNICELLI

*Director, Appleton Outpatient Clinic, McLean Hospital
and Associate Professor, Harvard Medical School*

THE GUILFORD PRESS
New York   London

© 1992 The Guilford Press
A Division of Guilford Publications, Inc.
72 Spring Street, New York, NY 10012

Printed in the United States of America

This book is printed on acid-free paper

Last digit is print number: 9 8 7 6 5 4 3 2 1

Library of Congress Cataloging-in-Publication Data

Vannicelli, Marsha.
    Removing the roadblocks : group psychotherapy with substance
abusers and family members / Marsha Vannicelli.
      p.   cm.   — (Guilford substance abuse series)
    Includes bibliographical references and index.
    ISBN 0-89862-174-7
    1. Substance abuse—Treatment.   2. Adult children of alcoholics—
Rehabilitation.   3. Group psychotherapy.   4. Psychodynamic
psychotherapy.   5. Family psychotherapy.   I. Title.   II. Series.
    [DNLM: 1. Family Therapy—methods.   2. Psychotherapy, Group—
methods.   3. Substance Abuse—therapy.   WM 270 V268r]
    RC564.V39   1992
    616.86'0651—dc20
    DNLM/DLC
    for Library of Congress   91-35427
                                                                        CIP

❖ *Foreword* ❖

From the beginning of what has been called the "alcoholism movement," group therapy has had an honored place in the array of treatments. As early as 1944, almost a half century ago, R. G. McCarthy (1946) began group therapy with alcoholic patients in an outpatient clinic. It was a moment, interestingly enough, when group therapy was considered to be an innovative and somewhat controversial method. Although psychiatry (at least in New Haven, where I was) was very much psychoanalytically oriented, the self-help movement had already begun and Alchoholics Anonymous was on its way. The clinic in which those early pioneering group sessions took place was the Yale Plan Clinic, which included a professional team of physician, social worker, psychologist, educator, and physiologist. This team maintained good working relations with the self-help movement; and, of the twenty patients who participated in those early sessions recorded by McCarthy, twelve were active in Alcoholics Anonymous. The sixteen sessions that took place were recorded in full, and it should be noted that in two of those sessions, spouses were invited and attended. There were fifteen men and five women in this early group—a ratio which, in terms of the alcoholic population, is probably still reasonably appropriate.

Although current audiovisual recording is more sophisticated in presenting ". . . restlessness or strained tension, alterations in facial expression, bursts of nervous laughter" (McCarthy, 1949), it is illuminating to read the comments of the group leader and to note that so many of the questions are still being asked today: Why does the alcoholic drink? What does alcohol do for the alcoholic? What are the troubles and the consequences associated with heavy drinking?

McCarthy presents to the group his view that, ". . . every alcoholic experiences discomfort . . . the feeling that life is threatening . . . a sense of restlessness" (McCarthy, 1949). A description of what the alcoholic experiences reminds us how far we have come from talk about "personality factors" (McCarthy's term). The heterogeneity of substance abusers, the modest advances in psychosocial research methodology, and the considerable advances in biomedical research constantly remind us that the etiology of alcoholism and substance abuse is complex and has biological, psychological, and sociocultural components (Zucker & Gomberg, 1986).

This book is about current work in group therapy with substance abusers and their family members. It might be subtitled, *"Everything You Wanted to Know About Group Therapy with Substance Abusers but Were Afraid to Ask."* It covers the problems and issues in setting up a group, how to help the group begin, defining the journey, and removing the roadblocks. It deals with groups for substance abusers and some of their recovery-related defenses, couples groups in which one or both partners are recovering substance abusers, and family groups. There are roadblocks to be dealt with in the group itself, within the individual patient, and within the therapist.

As with Vannicelli's prevous works, the book is an antidote to those easy how-to books which show not only how to become a therapist in ten easy lessons, but which often point out the road to good adjustment—with no reference at all to the relevant contributions of a small army of researchers. In contrast, this book provides a theoretical rationale, a psychodynamic perspective which involves modification of Yalom's (1975) interactional group therapy model. While listing alternative substance abuse models, e.g., disease model, adaptational model, self-medication model, the book modestly makes no attempt to debate the issues, but does take the position—now adopted by many behaviorist therapists—that total abstinence is the way to begin the work of breaking down drug abuse and drug dependency. At all points in this discussion and in the exposition of group therapy methods and problems throughout, references to research reports and to available data are cited. This kind of integration, teaching a treatment method by explication, while citing the sources and research work upon which the method is built, is much to be desired. Would that we had more clinicians trained in the scholarship of research!

Instead, over the past 40 years, therapists and researchers in the substance abuse field have increasingly gone their separate ways and communication has been minimal. Although some practitioners do, indeed, have an anti-intellectual, "keep it simple," attitude, many are genuinely interested in new ideas and new methods. Yet they are frequently let down by their research colleagues who leave them out of the process. Researchers all too often formulate their ideas without input from clinicians, have their ideas peer-reviewed (and funded) by fellow researchers, and present their findings and do their writing primarily for other members of the research community. This is unfortunate, since those who work directly with patients are frequently excellent obeservers who could offer useful hypotheses to those who would listen. Furthermore, practitioners often seek research-based input. Yet such integration between the clinical and research arenas is increasingly uncommon.

Only a handful of authors write practically and pragmatically for practitioners while indicating knowledge of the research literature. Vannicelli is one of those all-too-rare combinations whose writing combines both practicality and scholarship. Her work is rooted in and linked to theory and research findings. What is more, her work shows common sense. This combination of clinical practicality, scholarship, and sensibility was apparent as far back as the '70s when, during the "Great Sex-Role Debate," literature proliferated about sex-role changes, sexual indentity, and sexual strain and conflict, as explanations for the development of alcoholism among women. One report (hers) cut through the rhetoric:

> . . . our data indicate that sex-role *conflict*, rather than any particular sex-role stance or the extremity of the stance, is related to alcohol misuse . . . . Our data suggests further that focusing on sex-role orientation in absolute may be less productive than pursuing a direction-free model that focuses on *conflict* between levels or aspects of sexuality (Scida & Vannicelli, 1979, p. 41). (Italics mine)

Such clarity of thinking is a hallmark of the current book. Although I have not done group work with alcoholic patients, Vannicelli's work and her method of writing about it are so interesting and challenging that they inspire in the reader a desire to be trained in group work. The clinical materials (Database Outline, Face Sheet, Outpatient Psychotherapy Group Ground rules), the references, and the annotated bibliography only add to interest. And even if I am not ready to switch careers, to give up research for clinical work, the book inspires new dedication to the kind of applied research that is directed toward increasing knowledge about those who are willing to come in and to be helped.

Ann Arbor   EDITH S. LISANSKI GOMBERG, Ph.D
Michigan

❖ Preface ❖

Most books on group psychotherapy (and psychotherapy in general) describe clinical dilemmas, but tend to be extremely weak as practical guides for picking up the pieces (or avoiding the dilemmas in the first place). This book, however, is designed to help practitioners problem-solve and formulate appropriate strategies for thinking about their clinical work. Based on my experience over the past 18 years supervising group therapists in the addictions—individually, in dyads, and in large supervision groups—this volume addresses the dilemmas of everyday life in group psychotherapy, providing specific case material and suggestions not only for understanding the dilemmas, but working to resolve them, as well. Brought together in this single volume are the group therapy issues that arise for the three populations commonly treated in substance-abuse clinics (substance abusers, adult children of alcoholics, and other family members). I address the overlap among these three populations in terms of basic procedures, format, and hurdles that the leaders face, as well as suggesting special issues unique to each population.

I address these dilemmas from a psychodynamic perspective—using a modified version of Yalom's (1975) interactional group psychotherapy model that integrates some of the psychodynamic group perspectives of Rutan and Stone (1984). Although theory is not emphasized, clinical material, therapeutic strategies, and techniques are understood and explained within this theoretical framework.

The therapeutic model described is basically intended for long-term psychotherapy groups with outpatients. However, many of the roadblocks that are highlighted (in the group, in the individual patient, and in the therapist) are similar to those encountered in inpatient groups, even in groups that have relatively rapid turnover; and the reader who is running these groups will find much that is applicable. In addition, the basic model has been used in our clinic, with some modification, for more time-limited groups. Although leaders are more active in short-term groups and structure group interactions to attend more clearly to the group's focus (be that a short-term substance-abuse group, a family-members group, or an ACOA group), most of the dilemmas that the therapist faces apply to these short-term groups as well as to the long-term therapy groups that form the frame of reference for this text.

Throughout the book I have included many clinical examples and, wherever possible, a statement of the rationale for my interventions. This is intended to help the practitioner readily identify what from her past clinical experience is generalizable to her work with substance abusers and family members, and what may be new or may need to be modified. I pay special attention to the therapeutic stance—where the therapist positions herself with regard to the patient and why—and how various strategies and techniques aid in maintaining a consistent stance that will maximize the patient's opportunities for therapeutic growth. In addition, I give special attention to countertransference and the ways it can be used productively to facilitate the therapeutic work. Considerable attention is also paid to the therapeutic contract as a vehicle for setting a framework for the work, examining deviations, and understanding the course of the therapy.

This book does not attempt to settle, or even to comprehensively review, the many complicated questions about substance abuse that remain topics of hot debate among practitioners in the field. Nor does the group therapy model described require that the therapist choose between a disease model of substance abuse (Jellinek, 1960) and a psychological/adaptational model based on social learning theory (Marlatt, 1985; Miller, 1983) or self-medication theory (Khantzian, Halliday, & McAuliffe, 1990; Cooper, 1987). This book does, however, strongly endorse the view that treatment for substance abusers will proceed most effectively when a philosophy of total abstinence is embraced. Notwithstanding current debate, controversy, and considerable evidence on *both* sides regarding the possibility that some substance abusers who are not physiologically dependent might, under some circumstances, be effectively trained to use their substance of choice in moderation,* my own clinical experience both in my private practice and in the clinic that I have directed for 18 years is that at least for the population of patients that is coming to us for treatment, abstinence is still the soundest platform on which to begin the clinical work. This is consistent with my own view, shared by many others in the substance-abuse field (Vaillant et al., 1983; Washton, 1989; Weisman & Robe, 1983; Zimberg, 1982), that the patient's continued abuse of substances compromises his ability to work on other issues. Thus, while he is actively using, and as long as concerns about use predominate, this is our first order of business (not so different from the approach we might take with the patient whose ability to work on his issues is compromised by some other form of seriously self-destructive behavior).

Recognizing that therapists who are drawn to working with substance abusers and their family members range widely in terms of their professional backgrounds, extent of training, and credentials—with licensed professionals as well as many paraprofessionals drawn to this work—this book is aimed at four major populations of therapists:

1. Dynamically oriented professionals in the mental health field who have already had experience doing group psychotherapy with other populations and wish to apply their group psychotherapy expertise to their work with substance abusers and family members. These readers will already have a basic understanding of the ways in which the past influences current behavior and perceptions and will have some familiarity with the interactional group psychotherapy model of Yalom (1975).

2. Trained professionals who are currently treating substance abusers and/or their family members in individual therapy and are interested in exploring the possibility of expanding their practice to include dynamically oriented group psychotherapy for these populations as well.

3. Therapists, both individual and group, at all levels of training

---

* Miller (1983) argues that were there more programs that did not have an abstinence orientation, more patients—probably those in earlier phases of substance abuse—might present for treatment, and that our experience with these patients might alter our thinking about the abstinence model.

who are interested in better understanding common road-blocks in the therapist that impede the therapeutic journey. In particular, these readers will have an opportunity to explore the ways in which countertransference issues influence their work with clients and the ways in which understanding one's own countertransference reactions can enhance the therapeutic work.

4. Paraprofessional counselors, who will find many sections of the book relevant to their work with substance abusers and family members (even if they are not yet adequately trained to do psychodynamically oriented group psychotherapy) and who may be thinking about further training in the mental health field more generally, and group psychotherapy in particular.

In writing this second volume I have had to make a series of decisions about how much of the material that I covered in my first text (Vannicelli, 1989) would be repeated in the second. On the one hand, I felt that the second book, like the first, should stand on its own so that a reader who picked up either volume would have the essentials for starting and maintaining a group. On the other hand, since there will no doubt be readers who will read both books, I was not happy about repeating the same material. Neither the solution of assuming that this book should stand on its own nor the solution of assuming that most readers would have gotten all the essentials from the first book seemed appropriate. Thus, I decided to compromise: I have repeated all of the essentials relating to initiating the group, setting the group contract, and countertransference issues to which the leader must pay special attention. However, to minimize redundancy, whenever possible I have used new clinical examples. For less essential material, I have simply referred the reader to the previous volume in which a given issue was discussed more fully.

I begin (Chapter 1) with an introduction that describes the clinical populations of interest and their increasing awareness regarding the need for treatment. Chapter 2 discusses the rationale for group psychotherapy with these populations—describing some of the specific ways in which a dynamically oriented therapy group can be helpful. In Chapter 3, the reader is given an opportunity to consider some of the issues involved in setting up a group and selecting and preparing members. Chapter 4 deals with the actual beginning of a group. Chapter 5 focuses on special population issues for substance abusers, ACOAs, and other collaterals of substance abusers that affect the course of the group work. Chapter 6 defines the therapeutic journey that group leaders and group members will embark upon. Chapters 7, 8, 9, and 10 explore roadblocks or resistances—in the group (Chapter 7), the patient (Chapters 8 and 9), and the leader (Chapter 10)—that may impede the work and suggest ways of maneuvering around these inevitable roadblocks. Chapter 11 addresses the training and preparation of the group therapist from the standpoint of both the alcohol- and drug-related content areas important for his effectiveness and specific group psychotherapy training. Finally, the conclusion (Chapter 12) examines future directions and research considerations.

Acknowledgments

Many wonderful people have made execution and completion of this book possible.

My mentor and friend, Howard Blane, Ph.D. has been a continuous source of support. Many other friends and colleagues have also generously given their time and critical input: Geraldine Alpert, Ph.D., who found no clinical or editorial issue too large or too small to thoughtfully tackle; Dale Dillavou, Ph.D., Sharon Greenfield, Psy.D., Steven Tottingham, M.S.W., John Rodolico, Ph.D., Paul Simeone, Ph.D., Robert Jampel, Ph.D., and Melissa Shaak, Ed.M., all of whom provided clinical wisdom and editorial input; and David Schreier, B.A., who took interest in every aspect of the book from style and content to aspects of production.

In addition, the team of support staff at the Appleton Outpatient Clinic has been consistently helpful: in particular, Regina Roberts, Office Manager, who made the book an office priority and involved herself personally in its execution at many turns, and Chris Hache, who extended herself in many ways to assist in its completion. I am especially grateful to my transcriber, Dot Kimball, who always seemed to know exactly what I meant (even when my words were not so clear), and whose consistent enthusiasm for the project kept me productively writing in order to keep her happily occupied.

I owe special thanks to Alan Marlatt, Ph.D. and the Psychology Department of the University of Washington, Seattle, whose generosity and hopitality during my visiting professorship provided a stimulating and peaceful environment in which to complete this manuscript.

In addition, my gratitude is extended to the many clinicians I have supervised over the years, whose questions have helped me to clarify the issues that we all struggle with. I am also grateful to their patients, as well as my own, since it is the journeys that they invite us to take with them that continuously challenge us to clarify our thinking.

❖ *Contents* ❖

8. REMOVING THE ROADBLOCKS WITHIN THE PATIENT 138

❖ REMOVING THE ROADBLOCKS ❖
Group Psychotherapy with Substance Abusers and Family Members

❖ *1* ❖
Introduction

There has been a growing awareness in the past decade of the impact of substance abuse, not only on the substance abuser but on family members as well. This is documented by a 1990 Gallup Poll in which 23% of respondents indicated that drinking had been a cause of trouble in their family—a 20% increase over the affirmative response rate of a survey only 1 year earlier, and double the response rate obtained in a similar survey in 1974 (Gallup & Newport, 1990). Recent data regarding adult children of alcoholics (ACOAs) suggest similar increases in awareness of the familial impact of alcoholism, with 15 ACOA meetings registered with Al-Anon World Headquarters in New York in 1981 and 1,900 registered in 1989 (Collet, 1990).* However, public awareness gives only part of the picture.

The fuller picture includes data reflecting the numbers of individuals and family members who are adversely affected by substance abuse. In this book, "substance abuse" refers to the use of mood-altering drugs to the detriment of the user's interpersonal or occupational functioning or his physical or emotional well-being. Such mood-altering drugs include alcohol, prescription drugs (stimulants, sedatives, tranquilizers, analgesics), cocaine, heroin, marijuana, and a variety of other street drugs including hallucinogens and inhalants—chemical substances which are more and more frequently being used in combination.† Best estimates of actual prevalence figures for alco-

---

*In addition, by 1989 another 1,300 meetings were registered with the West Coast ACA group, which broke away from Al-Anon in 1984 (Collet, 1990).

†It is not the purpose of this book to focus on therapy groups for those who abuse nicotine or caffeine, although therapists who lead groups that focus on achieving abstinence from these drugs will find applicable many of the principles and strategies described.

holism suggest that 11–16% of the adult population in the United States (using overall lifetime prevalence rates) meet DSM-III criteria for alcohol abuse or dependence (Robins et al., 1984). Best estimates regarding prevalence of drug abuse (other than alcohol) suggest that 5–6% of the population will, at some point in their lives, experience drug abuse or drug dependence (Robins et al., 1984), with a conservative estimate of 550,000 Americans who may be at significant risk for experiencing problems from their use and abuse of cocaine (Kozel & Adams, 1985) and an estimated 500,000 heroin abusers (Kaufman, 1985). Overall, an estimated 15–18% of the population will exhibit a dependence or abuse problem with alcohol or drugs at some point in their lives (Robins et al., 1984).*

Prevalence figures for the offspring of alcoholics and other drug abusers are more poorly documented, but it is estimated that there are some 22 million people in the United States today who are the grown offspring (age 18 or older) of parents who had alcohol problems (Russel, Henderson, & Blume, 1985) and 6.6 million younger offspring (under the age of 18). The number of offspring of other drug abusers is also considerable (although solid estimates are more difficult to obtain, given the relative recency of large numbers of illicit drug abusers of childbearing age and the more hidden nature of prescription drug abuse in adults of childbearing age). However, in the coming years, we will undoubtedly be treating more and more of the by-products (offspring) of the past decade's increase in drug abuse.

Yet even when we add the available prevalence data to the data regarding increasing awareness, it is still difficult to clearly estimate the toll of substance abuse on substance abusers themselves, on their family members, and on the rest of society. As Steinglass, Bennett, Wolin, and Reiss (1987) point out, the alcoholism literature suggests that the negative impact is considerable. These authors cite several studies linking a formidable list of behaviors to alcohol use: spouse and child abuse (Hindman, 1979), divorce (Schuckit & Morrisey, 1976), depression and suicide (Winokur, 1974, 1979; Woodruff, Guze, Clayton, & Carr, 1973), and occupational problems (Berry, Boland, Smart, & Kanak, 1977). Yet, as Steinglass also points out, "although alcoholism often appears as a coincident condition and hence is correlated

---

*Although *use* does not necessarily constitute abuse, population estimates of use from a national population survey (NIDA, 1989) are included in Appendix A.

with such problems as family violence and suicide, there is little solid evidence that these factors are *causally* linked" (italics are my own). Moreover, he points to the number of families that "seem to be 'making do' despite having an alcoholic member in their midst" (p. 23).

In citing Steinglass' conclusions, it is not my intention (nor was it his) to downplay in any way the significant negative consequences of substance abuse for the substance abuser or for her family. Rather, it is to move the focus from an emphasis on the dramatic, often horrific coincident conditions (which may or may not be causally linked to substance abuse) and to focus on the often less dramatic but very real *pain* that we see in all those who present for treatment related to their own or a family member's substance abuse. Sometimes the exact nature of the pain for family members (and even for the substance abuser herself) is not altogether clear.* As Steinglass points out, reviewing a 1979 survey by NIAAA of adult drinking practices (Clark & Midanik, 1982), "respondents were hard pressed to point to specific family-related adverse effects associated with excessive drinking, although again, the numbers of people reporting problem drinking were very high. Thus, once again the 'ache' is there, but the attempt to localize the pain is unsuccessful" (p. 24). It is my view that attending to the "ache" forms the crux of our work as we treat substance abusers and their family members. Often a significant part of our task is to help our patients more clearly articulate and understand their pain in order to enable them to modify their lives in ways that will ease it.

In focusing on the pain, I break somewhat with tradition in the substance-abuse field by putting less emphasis on labels and diagnostic categories and more emphasis on heterogeneity within categories and each individual's uniqueness. As Yalom (1990) so elegantly states, "even the most liberal system of psychiatric nomenclature does violence to the being of another. If we relate to people believing that we can categorize them, we neither identify nor nurture the parts, the vital parts, of the other that transcends category" (p. 185). In keeping with this, I have dispensed with the detailed diagnostic descriptions com-

---

*Research suggests that in a myriad of ways the physical (as well as emotional) health of both substance abusers and their family members may be seriously compromised, with general health costs at least 100% greater for untreated alcoholics and their families than for nonalcoholics and their families—costs that are significantly reduced by treatment (Holder, 1987).

mon in introductory chapters of books on substance abuse—descriptions that differentiate specific categories of substance abuse with precise DSM-III* definitions detailing the characteristic symptoms associated with abuse of each kind of chemical substance as well as the distinctions between substance *abuse* and substance *dependence.* Such distinctions and categorizations, while helpful initially in assessing the nature and magnitude of the patient's substance-abuse problems, recede in usefulness once we begin the work of psychotherapy. As I am getting to know a patient, either in individual therapy or in group, I am not treating "an alcoholic," a "coke addict," "an ACOA," or a "co-dependent." Rather, I am working with a person in pain who hopes to trust me enough to permit me to enter her world and understand it with her.

In keeping with my disinclination toward labels, I do not insist that a substance abuser begin treatment by labeling herself "alcoholic" or "addicted." The patient and I need to agree that there is a problem around substance use, that we are going to address this first and foremost, and that this problem is part and parcel of other problems that will be addressed in our work together. Similarly, my work with the patient does not require that either she or I have made a definitive decision about whether the substance abuse has caused the other problems or vice versa. What is important is the patient's recognition that the substance abuse is part of the picture and that her many problems (including substance abuse) are inextricably interwoven. We assume neither that when the substance abuse is addressed that all of the other problems will disappear nor that when the other problems are addressed that the substance abuse problem will disappear. Each needs to be respected in its own right if the patient is to grow.

As the reader proceeds through this book, he will notice a linguistic thrust to my interventions that emphasizes the patient's strengths and potential for growth. The view that is reflected throughout is that our patients do the best they can, and the ineffectual strategies that they embrace were learned because at some point they were adaptive. People come to us for help when the solutions of the past no longer work. Our job is to help them understand where the old solutions came from, how they now get in the way, and how to find new

---

Diagnostic and Statistical Manual (third edition) of the American Psychiatric Association (1987), currently used for defining clinical diagnosis.

solutions that will be more effective. In keeping with a focus on the patient's adaptations and strengths, I also break with the common tradition in this field of focusing on "denial." I do so not because I believe that substance abusers and their family members do not use denial as a defense, but rather, because I believe it is more useful to think about the *many* defensive adaptations these patients use that are, in most ways, not so very different from the kinds of defensive adaptations used by most people in pain.*

This book describes the use of group psychotherapy as a vehicle for removing the roadblocks that so often keep our patients from getting past their pain. It pays special attention to roadblocks in the patient and in the therapist that need to be removed if the patient is to get the help that she needs. But perhaps a few words are also in order about cultural roadblocks in the therapeutic community that have historically blocked the effective treatment of substance abusers, thus adversely affecting the well-being of their family members as well.

When I began my own clinical work in the substance-abuse field nearly 20 years ago, treating alcoholics in groups, I had had positive group experience with other populations using the basic model described by Yalom (1970), and I was taken with the power of the therapy group for creating change. Not having been exposed at that point to the prevailing bias *against* dynamically oriented work with alcoholics—the view that alcoholics cannot tolerate the anxiety of insight-oriented treatment (Alexander, 1948; Gordis, 1987; Wolberg, 1948)—I and the staff that I supervised at the Appleton Outpatient Clinic began our own groups, fully expecting positive outcomes. In retrospect, I believe that our positive expectations were crucial to our success.

Since many people at that time believed that dynamically oriented group work (or, for that matter, dynamically oriented treatment of any kind) could not be done with alcoholics, my colleagues and I have given considerable thought to trying to understand both the origins of this view and the source of its perpetuation (Vannicelli, Dillavou, & Caplan, 1988). From the side of the psychiatric community, one can well imagine that the bias grew out of the frustrations and negative experiences of practitioners who attempted to use traditional therapy

---

*Miller (1983), in an extensive review of literature pertinent to the issue of denial, has found consistent evidence that alcoholics and other drug abusers are no more inclined to use denial than are other clinical populations.

on alcoholic patients who continued to drink. These practitioners neither understood the importance of abstinence to the patient's ability to do dynamically oriented work nor had the skills to help patients become abstinent. Many such therapists sat for years with patients who continued to drink and to benefit minimally from therapy. As traditional therapists became disenchanted with their ability to help this population, alcoholic patients, in turn, became disenchanted with the treaters who seemed to do so little that was helpful. Dynamically oriented therapists came to reject the alcoholic as a suitable patient—a rejection that was matched by the alcoholic community's discouragement with the traditional therapist. Years of uninformed treatment by dynamically oriented therapists had created a situation in which both the alcoholic community and the therapeutic community felt that dynamically oriented work could be of little use to this population.

This bias on the part of dynamically oriented caregivers (extended more generally to their feelings about treating many kinds of substance abuse) is not uncommon even today. What is most interesting about this is that it is common even among therapists who do use dynamically oriented therapy with other self-destructive, crisis-prone populations (e.g., adolescent or suicidal patients). What these dynamically oriented treaters have correctly understood is that exploratory, interpretive work may not be appropriate during the peak of a self-destructive crisis. During such times, the patient needs to be supported and contained until restabilized. However, once the crisis has passed, the exploratory work can resume.

Yet clinicians have been reluctant to view alcohol- and drug-related behaviors in similar ways. Instead of seeing the drinking or drug use as a period of crisis for the patient in which supportive, containing mechanisms are appropriate, these patients are often viewed in a globally negative way. Thus, the alcoholic or drug abuser is seen as a "crisis-prone, acting-out individual," also often described in terms such as "immature" or "inadequate." It is likely that these kinds of feelings and attitudes about substance abuse have to do with the treater's pessimism about whether this particular form of self-destructive behavior can be contained.

Our approach at the Appleton Outpatient Clinic (Griefen, Vannicelli, & Canning, 1985; Vannicelli, 1982, 1988; Vannicelli, Canning, & Griefen, 1984) is to pay careful attention to containing the substance abuse, to getting it specifically managed through the use of carefully negotiated stepwise contracts that add supports, as needed, for maintaining abstinence (including the use of AA, NA, Antabuse, naltrexone, and relapse-prevention training), and, alongside of this, to do dynamically oriented individual and group therapy once abstinence is relatively stabilized. It should be noted that we do not simply take active substance abusers and put them together in a group—a strategy that others have tried, with understandable failure. All patients placed in our long-term therapy groups have either had prior inpatient treatment (generally 2–4 weeks) followed by participation in an outpatient transition group for several weeks; or, if they begin with us as outpatients, they will have participated in several individual sessions in which contracting for abstinence begins, followed by participation (drug-free) in a 5-week, twice-weekly education and therapy sequence. Only once all this preparation is done are patients referred to long-term dynamically oriented groups.

It is my hope, as the reader proceeds through the chapters that follow, that I can transmit not only the clinical intervention strategies that we have found effective but also a sense of the enthusiasm and optimism, originally brought to my work through sheer naivete, that have been borne out and heightened by nearly 20 years of experience doing group psychotherapy with these populations.

❖ 2 ❖
Rationale for Dynamically Oriented Group Psychotherapy

Group psychotherapy has long been an essential component of alcohol- and drug-treatment programs. Although group orientations vary based on setting and population (Blume, 1985; Brix, 1983; Brown & Beletsis, 1986; Brown & Yalom, 1977; Brunner-Orne, 1956; Cermak & Brown, 1982; Cooper, 1987; Doroff, 1977; Elder, 1990; Fox, 1962; Honig & Spinner, 1986; Igersheimer, 1959; Khantzian et al., 1990; Perez, 1986; Sands & Hanson, 1971; Scott, 1963; Seixas & Levitan, 1984; Steiner, 1977; Vannicelli, 1982, 1987, 1989, 1990; Washton, 1989; Yalom, 1974), professionals seem to agree that group work offers substance abusers and their family members unique opportunities: (1) to share and to identify with others who are going through similar problems, (2) to understand the impact of alcohol and drugs in their lives and the defenses that keep them adversely entangled with chemical substances (and/or with those who abuse these substances), (3) to learn more about their own and others' feelings and reactions, and (4) to learn to communicate needs and feelings more directly.

The group model that forms the frame of reference for this book is basically the dynamic interactional therapy model, which has been described in detail by Yalom (1975). In weekly 90-minute sessions, 8 to 10 members, in a state of personal distress, come together with a number of strangers. They are dissimilar from one another except for the shared status of being patients in a therapy group and, in the case of special population groups such as those described here, their shared presenting issues (substance abuse problems, ACOA issues, etc.). There is an expectation that members will share personal things about themselves—their thoughts, feelings, or behavior—that are ordinarily considered private. Personal self-disclosure in this unique situation creates a sense of initial cohesiveness and similarity among members, along with the feeling that participants are different from others outside of the group.* In this unique group context the 11 curative factors outlined by Yalom,† come into play as members explore their interpersonal relationships within the group. Group members are encouraged to explore in depth their style of relating to the leader(s) and other members by interacting freely and honestly in the immediate present while at the same time assuming a self-reflective pose. The group is seen as a special social microcosm in which basic feelings and life themes replay themselves and can be worked through. The group's task is to help members better understand and alter self-defeating ways of relating so that more meaningful relationships can be established.

Our approach is similar to the Stanford group therapy model used for substance abusers (Yalom, 1974;, Brown & Yalom, 1977) and for ACOAs (Cermak & Brown, 1982; Brown & Beletsis, 1986). However, the group model that we use differs from the model described by Yalom and Brown and their colleagues in three respects that make it more similar to the psychodynamic group therapy model described by Rutan and Stone (1984). First, leaders do not provide the written group summaries used by Brown and Yalom (1977) in their work with substance abusers and by Cermak and Brown (1982) in their work with ACOAs. Second, more emphasis is placed on the group leader's understanding of his own feelings and reactions (countertransference) as a way of understanding important issues in the group as well as important roadblocks. Finally, more attention is given to group-as-a-whole dynamics within the group (Bion, 1961).

In terms of practical applications, our approach also has much in common with the model recently articulated by Khantzian et al. (1990) in their work with cocaine abusers. However, in contrast to their assumption that preexisting characterological deficits underlie the

---

*Lieberman (1983) reviews research that he has done along with colleagues, documenting the relationship between these group characteristics and the groups' perceived helpfulness.

†(1) Instillation of hope, (2) universality, (3) imparting of information, (4) altruism, (5) the corrective recapitulation of the primary family group, (6) development of socializing techniques, (7) imitative behavior, (8) interpersonal learning, (9) group cohesiveness, (10) catharsis, (11) existential factors.

substance abuse (and that specific deficits lead to particular drug choices), we make no universal assumptions about the causal direction of the relationship between the patient's substance abuse and his other problems.

Advantages of Group Psychotherapy

We view this kind of group therapy as a particularly helpful modality for substance abusers and their family members, and often the treatment of choice, for a number of reasons that are elaborated in the sections that follow. In addition, in terms of cost-effectiveness, group has much to recommend it, particularly in this day of the shrinking health-care dollar. The charge for 90 minutes of group psychotherapy is generally one-half to one-third the cost of 50 minutes of individual therapy. This cost data is even more persuasive given the considerable research data on treatment outcome for substance abusers that generally point to results that are at least as favorable for group psychotherapy as for individual psychotherapy (Brandsma & Pattison, 1985; Emrick, 1975; Kanas, 1982; Solomon, 1983).

Reducing the Sense of Isolation

The grouping together of people who have identified themselves as having a problem in common (substance abusers or ACOAs or family members living with a chemically dependent relative) provides an initial sense of shared experience, thus increasing the possibility for initial bonding. As Yalom points out in his discussion of "universality," "Many patients enter therapy with a disquieting thought that they are unique in their wretchedness" and the disconfirmation of these feelings of uniqueness can be a powerful source of relief (p. 7). The group thus presents at least the possibility of belonging and of being understood.

Instilling Hope

The group provides an opportunity for members to see others who are getting better. Members often experience a sense of hope when others in the group talk, in the past tense, of problems that they are currently facing—communicating that these problems are something that they have known *in the past* but have now worked through. This is one advantage of an open-ended group in which new members join as older members graduate and members are at different stages in their treatment. However, even in a group where all participants are in the early phases of treatment, members will work through different problems at different rates and can thus provide areas of hope for one another.

Conversely, hope can also be instilled by the opportunity to judge one's own progress against the yardstick of others who are still stuck. It is not unusual to hear a patient reflect, upon listening to a newcomer in the group, "Hey, doesn't that sound familiar? Remember how I used to get stuck in that rut?"

Learning from Watching Others

The opportunity to watch other members in action who are struggling with similar kinds of conflicts is often useful in giving a clear view of the ways in which others get stalled at critical points. There is thus an opportunity to understand dysfunctional behavior and aborted communications by watching them being played out in the group.

Even during "rest periods" when patients are not actively grappling with their own problems, important growth may occur while they are processing the work of others. This paradoxical "rest" is especially likely when issues that are being defended against in the "resting" member are being actively processed by another, thus giving the resting (defended) member an opportunity to gain vicariously as the other works. It is often the case, in fact, that a patient who is defending against her own problems may eagerly engage in helping another sort out issues that are closely related—not recognizing until later the relevance to her own experience as well.

Equally important, members model for one another useful ways of communicating and interacting. By observing others, members thus have an opportunity to learn not only what does *not* work but also to get a first-hand view of *successful* interactions. The group provides a safe arena in which members can learn more about their own feelings and those of others and how their feelings can be most effectively communicated.

Learning by Acquiring Information

Group psychotherapy offers the opportunity for learning along a number of fronts and also for acquiring a considerable amount of information, not only about oneself but also about "what makes people tick."

As Yalom points out, by the conclusion of a successful interactional group therapy experience, most patients have learned a great deal about psychic functioning, the meaning of symptoms, interpersonal and group dynamics, and the process of psychotherapy itself. However, he also emphasizes that the educational process is an implicit one—not to be confused with the focus or intent of an education group. The therapist does not offer explicit didactic intervention. Rather, the questions that we ask and our clarifications and interpretations provide information that can further group members' understanding of themselves in relationship to others. For example, as Wood (1987) points out in her discussion of ACOAs, information about the effects of parental alcoholism is "frequently offered in the context of an interpretation, at a moment when a patient is or has recently been in the throes of an emotional conflict, so that a particular bit of information will likely elucidate the original source of the conflict" (p. 121).

This is nicely illustrated in a case example of a patient who had powerful wishes to "share his grief and fear" that were offset by equally powerful wishes to flee and to protect himself. Wood handled this by pointing out to the patient

> . . . that his struggles with his family around emotional sharing made his present struggle with himself quite understandable. I observed that alcoholic families frequently convey a powerful message to children that their needs for intimacy, support, and comfort are pathological, and I reassured him that, in fact, these feelings were a very human, and very valuable, part of him. (p. 139)

Altering Distorted Self-Concepts

Because of the potential in the group for examining one's own behavior in relation to others (and getting group feedback), members have an opportunity to discover ways in which their self-images have been distorted and the myths about themselves that continue to be perpetuated from the past. In addition, as members have an opportunity to identify with others and to accept them in spite of their flaws and secrets, they also learn to be more accepting of these characteristics in themselves. As such, the group experience provides a healthy climate for the special sense of comfort that comes from seeing oneself and others in perspective.

Reparative Family Experience

Group therapy also offers the possibility of a reparative family experience. Patients come to group therapy with histories of complicated and often unsatisfactory experiences in their first and most important group, the family of origin. As Yalom (1975) points out, the therapy group resembles a family in many ways, and members interact with one another and with the leaders in a manner characteristic of their past interactions with siblings and parents. Thus, the long-term interactional therapy group provides an immediate "family context" in which to explore the past as it is recreated in the present. In this new "family context" not only will early conflicts be recapitulated but the group provides an opportunity for them to be relived correctively" as nonadaptive behavioral patterns from the past are challenged and testing out of new behaviors is encouraged. Through this mechanism one not only has the opportunity to see one's family and one's role in it in greater perspective, but new and healthier ways of relating are also learned.

Aspects of Special Appeal for Specific Populations

Substance Abusers Groups

For substance abusers, group psychotherapy offers an additional advantage. Even when the patient is not in immediate danger with regard to his substance abuse, coming to a weekly substance abuse group keeps the issue alive. The opportunity to hear other people's concerns about (or difficulties with) abstinence underscores the need for constant vigilance. This is different in many ways from what happens in individual therapy. In individual therapy, particularly if it is relatively traditional therapy, the patient sets the agenda and largely determines what will be discussed. Weeks or months may go by in which the issue of substance abuse never comes up. Thus, individual therapy does not serve as the same kind of reminder as participation in a substance-abuse group. One could argue that an actively involved member of a 12-step program who is also in individual therapy might be able to achieve the same goal. Although to some extent this is so, often when patients begin to waver in their commitment to abstinence, they also slip away from AA and NA. Since AA does not require the same kind of accountability as a therapy group, early warning signs may not be noticed.

Family Members and ACOA Groups

Group therapy may also appeal to the ACOA and to other relatives of substance abusers for an additional reason that is quite distinct from the therapeutic value of group for these populations. Initially the family group and the ACOA group may appear to provide a forum in which members will be able to *externalize* the source of their discomfort and pain by focusing on their substance-abusing relatives. Thus, the family member's alcohol or drug problem provides what appears to be a single clear enemy and a specific thing to blame. For many ACOAs and other relatives of substance abusers, the idea that something outside of themselves is bad and needs to be attended to is an easier focus on which to begin therapy. Although this notion, if unchallenged, will ultimately interfere with the therapeutic work and will need to be addressed by the therapist (as discussed in Chapter 5) for people who have too long blamed themselves, this shift in focus may provide a source of initial relief.

Relationship of Group Psychotherapy to Self-Help Groups

Millions of substance abusers and their family members have found self-help groups (AA, NA, Al-Anon, Nar-Anon) to be an invaluable source of support. Membership in a self-help program often occurs alongside of membership in a psychotherapy group, and work in the two can be mutually complementary. Though many substance abusers, ACOAs, and other family members find that the support they receive in their self-help programs adequately addresses their issues, a psychotherapy group led by a trained professional offers a different kind of help. A leaderless group in which all members are participating, with the goal of self-help, has a very limited capacity to examine shared fallacies, group myths, and various kinds of intermember and group transference phenomena. In particular, the kinds of interpersonal issues that are detailed in Chapter 8, which are often so important in understanding how the past is being relived in the present, are difficult to work through (let alone objectively observe) in a leaderless self-help group.

Since many patients entering a psychotherapy group will have had prior experience in some kind of self-help group, it is important to clearly differentiate these two kinds of experiences, particularly the ways in which the expectations and ground rules differ, before bringing the patient into the group. These distinctions are detailed further in Chapter 3.

This chapter has described some of the ways in which group therapy can be helpful to substance abusers and their family members by reducing one's sense of isolation, instilling hope, and providing an opportunity both to learn from watching others and to alter distorted self-perceptions. Group therapy also provides a unique opportunity to create a "family context" in which the past can be explored as it is recreated in the present. The special advantages of group psychotherapy specific to groups for substance abusers and for family members have also been discussed, including the opportunities for growth distinct from those available in AA, Al-Anon, or other self-help groups. Now that we have reviewed some of the advantages of these groups for the members, the next chapter examines some of the issues that the potential leader must consider before deciding to begin a therapy group.

❖ *3* ❖
Considerations in Setting Up a Group: Selecting and Preparing Members

There are a number of issues to be considered in setting up a therapy group. First, the therapist must consider the structure and composition of the group—whether it will be a private practice or a clinic group, whether it will be time-limited or open-ended, whether group members will be seen by the therapist in individual therapy either before entering the group or concomitantly, and the degree of heterogeneity of group membership in terms of demographic characteristics and stage of recovery. Potential members need to be carefully screened in terms of alcohol and drug history, appropriateness for the group (in terms of motivation, staying power, and level of functioning), and in terms of the strain they may place on the existing group members. Pregroup interviews provide an opportunity not only to assess these dimensions but also to shape the patient's expectations regarding group participation.

Group Structure and Composition

Private Practice versus Clinic Group

Clinic groups, particularly if they are provided within the structure of an organized substance-abuse treatment program (such as the one diagrammed schematically in Appendix B), provide many advantages both for the clinician delivering services and for the patient. Backup services are generally more available (services for psychological testing, legal consultation, psychopharmacology consults, etc.), as are greater options for organized ancillary services for clients (individual, couples, and family therapy) along with the group treatment. Clinic groups may also offer the leader a greater opportunity for sharing with colleagues and for supervision (peer or otherwise). In addition, in a clinic group, backup coverage is often provided when the therapist must be away, and there is readily available emergency backup for admitting patients in need of hospitalization.

Generally in clinics a larger network of groups is available, not only facilitating patient match in terms of level of functioning but also providing more ready placement of patients who may present with one substance-abuse-related issue (e.g., the pain of living with a substance-abusing husband) but who may, in fact, have a more pressing substance-abuse issue (for example, her own problem with substance abuse). In a clinic patients can also be "contained" in a system that allows them the possibility of moving from one therapy group to another should their circumstances change (for example, a relatively low-functioning patient whose level of functioning improves after several months of psychopharmacological treatment can be readily moved to a higher-functioning group; similarly, the patient who comes in to work on her ACOA issues but whose substance-abuse problem later becomes apparent can be given a substance- abuse group along side of, or instead of, the ACOA group). Although none of these possibilities is ruled out in private practice, the private group therapist's understandable investment in continuing with a given patient and unfamiliarity or lack of connection to other available resources may pose obstacles to modifying the treatment plan when the patient's situation changes.

Other differences between the private practice model and the clinic model have to do with how patients are referred and how much information the group leader has about a patient prior to her initial meeting with him. Typically, in a clinic model, by the time the group therapist meets with the patient, an intake worker has already taken a thorough alcohol and drug history as well as a psychosocial history. This is less likely to be the case in private practice, where patients are more likely to call the group therapist directly to ask about a particular group that they have heard about. The group leader in private practice must decide how much information she needs to get from the patient (assuming there is not a referring person who can provide information) and, accordingly, how much time to spend on initial history taking and evaluation. Although I lean, both in our clinic and in my own private practice, to several pregroup interviews, this leaves open the question of what specific information the group therapist needs to have before accepting a patient into her group.

An adequate alcohol and drug history (discussed in a later section) is essential for all patients, particularly so for those who present for treatment because of their own or someone else's use of substances. In clinics this is generally provided before the pregroup interviews. The group leader in private practice will need to attend to this in some detail during the pregroup interviews. Generally in clinics a detailed psychosocial and developmental history is also part of the initial clinic record. Although many clinicians like having this information and find it useful to have prior to the patient's entry into the group, I generally find that the history that evolves during the course of the group work is sufficient when supplemented by a few focused questions about current and past significant connections. Thus, I ask briefly about the patient's connection to his family of origin and about current people with whom the patient is close. I also get some feeling for what the patient is involved with and committed to in both his personal and his work life (as well as what "goes wrong" in each of these areas). By so doing, I get a sense of the quality of his relationships, his ability to commit and connect, and his overall level of functioning.

Clearly, the therapist working in a clinic setting has a greater cushion of support and, in the ways discussed above, has more opportunity for collaboration, both in the initial referral of patients to his group and in terms of ongoing support, than does the therapist working in private practice. Groups in clinics tend to be somewhat less stressful for the therapist because of these supports. However, clinic groups are also generally less financially rewarding and may create complications for the group leader, including coordination with clinic schedules and somewhat less flexibility in terms of client selection.

Regardless of whether the group is initiated in one's private practice or in a clinic, issues regarding group size and composition, duration of the group, and whether time-limited or open-ended need to be addressed before member selection and screening actually begin. (The decision about whether one will have a co-therapist or not, and criteria for selecting a co-therapist, are also important to consider and are discussed in Chapter 10.)

The Use of Individual Therapy along with Group

For many patients, combining group and individual therapy optimizes the potential for growth. For some, individual therapy provides a safety net that makes it possible to tolerate and to explore in greater depth the powerful feelings that get stirred up in the group. For others, the group serves as a catalyst for the work of the individual therapy as conflicts are played out in the unique microcosm of the group. Possible variations include the following: (1) all members will be seen in individual therapy by the group leader (or one of the two leaders if co-led) along with participation in the group; (2) all members will be in individual therapy as well as the group but will be seen by therapists other than the group leader(s); (3) individual therapy will be optional, except in those cases in which the group leaders feel that individual therapy is essential along with membership in the group. Each of these possibilities has a different set of implications for group members and should be carefully considered prior to formation of the group.

If it is the group leader's wish that all members be seen in individual therapy along with the group, it is generally preferable that a decision be made in advance either that all patients will be seen by the leader (or co-leaders) of the therapy group or that none will be. When the leader sees some of the group members individually but not others, a situation is fostered in which some members truly have "special" status with regard to the leader(s). Concerns about who the leaders care most about, know the best, and are the most interested in are important issues in the life of the group. Providing a relatively uniform context in which either all patients are seen by the group leaders individually or none are establishes a cleaner screen on which to examine these issues.

Except in the situation in which all members are seen in individual therapy by the leader(s), extensive individual contacts with the leader(s) should generally be avoided. On the other hand, individual sessions may be necessitated for brief periods when a member is in a crisis of sufficient magnitude that the weekly group therapy sessions cannot sufficiently process and contain it. For brief periods (for example, one or two sessions), it may be useful for the group leader(s) to meet individually with the patient, with the understanding that the group knows about it and relevant information will be brought back into the group. As suggested above, if more extensive support is needed, it would generally be advisable for the patient to be referred to another individual therapist.

Although I prefer the "all-or-none" model with regard to group members being in individual therapy with the group leader(s), this ideal may not always be possible. If the leader does find that she needs to be involved individually in a more extensive way with a patient, and there seems to be no reasonable alternative, it is important that the group know about this and be encouraged to talk about their reactions to it. It is important that this occur not only when the therapist's "special relationship" with a group member begins but whenever it may be relevant throughout the course of the group.

Possible Pitfalls in Selecting Group Members from One's Own Caseload of Individual Therapy Patients

Although there may be many advantages to seeing the same patients both individually and in group therapy, it is important that the therapist be aware of some of the possible hazards of this situation. Patients who are already seeing the therapist individually, when invited to join the therapist's group, may feel pressured into it as a requirement for remaining in the therapist's good graces. This can be exacerbated further when a therapist decides to consolidate her practice by taking a certain number of patients and putting them together in a group *rather* than continuing to see them individually. These patients are placed in a peculiar dilemma. They may fear that if they refuse to go into the group, they will lose the therapist altogether. On the other hand, even if they do go into the group, there is still a considerable loss, since it is not the same to have the therapist all to oneself as it is to share her with six or seven other people.

It is important that the therapist be sensitive to the issues and concerns that may come up for the patient (often not fully explored or recognized by the therapist because of her own need to manage her caseload in a different way). Even if all the groundwork has been done in the individual sessions with each patient and it seems as if a viable group has been put together, lateness, no-shows, and canceled appointments early on may signal that the patient's feelings about the new treatment venture need to be more fully explored.

These kinds of problems are further intensified when the therapist has a relatively small number of patients to choose from for a given group and needs to have all or nearly all of them participate in order to make a go of the group (e.g., a therapist who decides to invite all of her ACOA patients to participate in a therapy group). If, in fact, she only has five such patients and needs all or most of them to agree to participate in order to proceed, it is difficult to imagine that these patients will not all feel a certain amount of pressure. The last few patients that the therapist talks to, after already getting an affirmative response from two or three others, may feel especially pressured. Selecting from one's own individual therapy caseload generally works better if the therapist either has a large enough caseload to select from or is in a position to allow plenty of time to talk about it with all of her patients—with the possibility of waiting to actually begin the group until new patients come into her practice. (This allows enough time to explore the issue without creating a sense of pressure.)

In a case that recently came to my attention, a therapist who was overworked and needed to consolidate her practice decided that she would take her five ACOA clients and put them together in a group instead of seeing them individually. Although all five of the patients did agree to participate, three did not show up the first night (two called with seemingly legitimate excuses, and the third simply no-showed). Of the remaining two who did show up, one called a few days after the session to say that the group had been "too upsetting" for her and that she did not think that she should continue. This is an example where all of the patients, given what seemed to be the only choice—to see the therapist in a group or not at all, *agreed* to participate. However, clearly, the issues had not been adequately worked through.

Open-Ended versus Time-Limited Groups

When beginning a new group it is also important to consider the advantages and disadvantages of open-ended versus time-limited groups. The open-ended group offers the advantages of long-term psychotherapy—allowing patients to stay as long as they need in order to work through their issues. It also, however, requires a long-term commitment on the part of the therapist who begins such a group. When first beginning to work with groups, leaders might want to consider a time-limited group, perhaps 6 months to a year, in which members begin together (or in near proximity) and end together on a specified date. If the group is time-limited, the group leader(s) should plan in advance the time frame during which new members will be added. Options include: (1) all members must be present the first night in order to join, (2) new members will be allowed to enter over the course of the first month, (3) the possibility of taking in new members will continue throughout the year. These options should be considered in advance, and group members should be told specifically what the operating ground rules will be. For example, though all members entering such a group will understand that they are expected to join the group for the entire course of the time-limited period, they should also be told what will happen if for some reason a member does drop out—that is, whether or not he will be replaced.

Group Composition: Demographic Heterogeneity

In putting together a new group (or in replacing departing members), it is important to keep in mind certain guidelines about group composition. In selecting members for groups, both in my clinic and in my private practice, I use the principle of "maximal tolerable heterogeneity." In my experience, the group functions best and has the most potential for a rich array of dynamics when there is diversity among members. Thus, even in a group that is homogeneous on a single important dimension (e.g., all are recovering substance abusers), whenever possible I lean toward a mixed-sex group that spans an age range of more than one generation (i.e., some members will be old enough to be other members' parents) in which there is also a mix in terms of socioeconomic backgrounds, defensive styles, and diagnoses. Often the greatest richness is created when a new member is brought in who complements the dynamics of another (possibly because of a generational issue) or who, despite socioeconomic differences, is working on an issue similar to the group's focus (e.g., around intimacy and partnering, or difficulties in separating).

While greater heterogeneity has a positive impact in terms of enhancing the richness of the group and making it possible to more easily integrate a greater variety of new members, there are limitations on heterogeneity that also must be considered. Thus, a single "outlier" should be brought into a group only after cautious reflection. For example, if a group consists of married and divorced members in their late 30s to late 40s, one should think seriously about placing an unmarried 22-year-old in such a group. If the leaders wish to diversify the group, they might consider bringing in two young unattached members so that neither would initially experience the sense of being all alone. Similarly, if a group has been composed of all female members and the leader wishes to make it a mixed-sex group, at least two men should be brought in. If one of the co-leaders is a male, it may be possible for a brief period of time to elapse before the second male member is introduced (but only if the entering male member is apprised in advance of his temporary outlier position).

Another limitation on heterogeneity relates to level of functioning of group members (Friedman, 1989). An unemployed, highly withdrawn patient recently discharged from the hospital would not be appropriately placed in a high-functioning group. Similarly, a high-powered executive, even if paired with another high-functioning member, would generally not be well suited to a group where most members were poorly functioning and still struggling to stabilize their work and personal lives. In my experience, however, leaders tend to err far more on the side of creating too much homogeneity than on the side of too much variation. Often, they are too cautious and protective of their groups, thereby restricting the group's potential vitality (as well as its ability to absorb future members).

In addition, if a patient believes that certain kinds of work cannot get done in a group that is mixed on certain dimensions, this may be an indication for placement in a more homogeneous group. For example, the ACOA patient who strongly identifies around her ACOA issues, feels that this is an essential focus, and also feels that she will be more comfortable in a group with other ACOAs in all likelihood will do better in a group with other ACOAs. After all, expectation for positive outcome is an important part of what makes for therapeutic growth. On the other hand, an ACOA who understands that her family-of-origin issues are important, but that they may overlap considerably with family-of-origin issues of people with different kinds of dysfunctional families, might do equally well in a more heterogeneous group. Similarly, the patient who believes she will not deal with certain kinds of issues in a mixed-sex group might do better with a referral to an all-women's group. Of course, in this case the gains to be had by greater initial comfort and more positive expectations regarding outcome need to be weighed against the limitations imposed on any group that cuts off a major portion of the population—e.g., all men (Alonso, 1987).

Finally, in substance-abuse groups, it is essential that all members are committed to working toward abstinence. The importance of a set of shared norms about what it means to be working on one's alcohol or drug problem should not be underestimated.* Although there is some disagreement about whether abstinence is the only appropriate goal for substance abusers, mixing patients with divergent goals in the same group poses an almost insurmountable challenge to the integrity of the group. Since the group members do not share a notion of what it means to get better, they find themselves at an impasse in terms of either helping one another to get there or assessing how they are doing. Furthermore, since the wish of nearly every recovering substance abuser is that he may some day be able to use alcohol or drugs again, the presence of a member in the group who is acting on this wish may well arouse anxiety that is dealt with by means of unproductive and extreme proselytizing (in support of AA, abstinence, etc.). For these reasons, the group leader, when initially selecting members and preparing them for entry into the group, should make it clear what the expectations are—namely, that all members will be working toward abstinence and that any difficulties encountered in working toward this goal (in the form of cravings, fears about drinking/drugging, or actual use) will be discussed with the group—and should be sure that potential members are willing to endorse a clear set of norms regarding substance use.

Mixing Patients with Varying Amounts of Sobriety: The Pro and Con of Therapy Groups Based on Stage of Recovery

Typically in substance-abuse treatment programs, aftercare groups for patients who have completed the intensive initial phase of treatment are based on one of two models—a stage-of-recovery model or a mixed-recovery model.

In the *stage-of-recovery model* separate groups are set up for patients in "early recovery" and for those patients who have been abstinent longer (usually at least 6 months). In this model, the early-recovery groups themselves may be time-limited (all patients beginning at a certain point and ending, for example, 6 months later). Once patients have finished their initial therapy commitment, they may move on individually to join a new longer-term group, or the group as a whole may recontract to become a long-term sobriety group. Or, alternatively, membership in the early-recovery group may be time-

---

*The initial elaboration of this idea can be found in Vannicelli (1982).

limited, but the group itself may go on indefinitely. Thus, each patient attends the early-recovery group for e.g., 6 months, but graduations and new arrivals are ongoing. (This variation is often more feasible for clinics in terms of the flow of patients.)

In the *mixed-recovery long-term therapy group model* patients join the group generally in early phases of recovery and continue as long as it is a productive therapeutic support for them. Membership is not time-limited and the number of months of recovery will vary considerably—with newer members generally having fewer months abstinent than older members. In such groups it is nearly impossible not to mix people in early recovery with those in later recovery, because people will be graduating from the group at their own pace and new members will need to come in. New members, almost invariably, are in earlier phases of recovery—usually looking for aftercare following management of the initial crisis phase of their treatment. Thus, long-term groups would find it very difficult to sustain themselves over time if they limited new members to those who were already abstinent for a considerable amount of time. The choice regarding these two options often depends on the fiscal management of the clinic. If the program aims to encourage patients to finish a piece of work in a time-limited period, with some opting to go on at the end of that time and others not, then the stage-of-recovery model is useful. In this model, most patients who join an "early recovery" group, upon "graduation," will not opt to go on. In programs that have a minimum amount of funding, this kind of time-limited service may be financially optimal. On the other hand, in programs in which there are no financial restraints regarding length of treatment, the mixed-recovery long-term model tends to be more common.

I prefer the mixed model for a number of reasons. First, mixing levels of abstinence provides a sense of optimism and hope to the newly recovering member. The fact that several people in the group have been there for a while and have been doing well—and even the fact that occasional slips can be "ridden out" without being totally detrimental—can provide a sense of tremendous hope for the new member who is worried about what recovery is going to bring. In addition, the definition of "early recovery" is not always clear. Some patients who have been "white-knuckling it" for the first 2 years of recovery may look very similar to others who are only 3 months into their recovery. Recovery is not a straight line path—patients move in and out of their "stage" of recovery. A person who has abstained for three years, even as AA conceptualizes it, is still only committed "one day at a time" to sobriety. Thus, when determining an individual's phase of recovery, I am less comfortable with a fixed time frame—for example, a specific number of months since last use of alcohol or drugs—than I am in thinking about how far the patient is from his preoccupation with these substances. Some patients decide to stop drinking, get supports in place, use these supports to deal with cravings and to avert crises that might otherwise have set off drinking, and within a few months of their last drink are able to move on to other aspects of their emotional growth. For others, during the first several months (or even years) after giving up alcohol and drugs, abstinence remains a primary preoccupation.

The mixed model has appeal precisely because psychological distance from substance abuse does wax and wane over time. Thus, a patient who has been abstinent 2 years may find himself facing the same kind of urges, following a major crisis, as someone earlier in recovery. And a member who is only a few weeks from his last drink may stir up issues that are alive in other members who have been abstinent for some time. A new, recently abstinent member, like an "old-timer" in the group who is actively grappling with fears about a slip, keeps alive for all members the importance of vigilance regarding substance abuse.

Member Selection and Prescreening

Going Beyond the Presenting Problem

Careful clinical assessment is an essential part of the work to be done before placing patients in therapy groups. Regardless of the particular presenting issue, it is important to know more about the patient—the severity of his presenting problems, concomitant problems, and his strengths as well as his troubled parts.

While the patient's self-diagnosis should be taken seriously, it should not get in the way of a more complete mental health assessment. For example, a substance abuser may present for treatment around his alcohol problem, unaware or unconcerned about his daily use of prescribed tranquilizers. Or the wife of a cocaine abuser may come for treatment seeking help coping with the strain placed on her by her husband's drug use, unaware that her own "occasional heavy partying with him" may need addressing. Similarly, a young woman may present for treatment around her ACOA issues who may be currently living with a chemically dependent person or who may be chemically dependent herself.*

Thus, in our clinic, where we have separate tracks (see diagram, Appendix B) for treating substance abusers, family members, and ACOAs, when an ACOA comes in for treatment around her ACOA issues, we confirm our interest in addressing these concerns. We also point out that we have learned that there are two other areas that are important to pay attention to from the outset—namely, that ACOAs frequently repeat the patterns of their past by marrying or settling in with a substance-abusing person or by having concerns about their own substance use.

If the intake therapist has concerns about the ACOA's current substance use, or if it is clear that the patient is currently living with an active user, the patient is introduced to the concept of "hierarchical treatment." This term is meant to express the idea that the problem of highest crisis potential is treated first, while at the same time careful attention is paid to the ACOA issue. If we do find that there is a substance-abuse problem, we tell the patient that we would like to treat this directly. She would then be referred to our clinic's substance-abuse track. We would also let her know that the ACOA problem would certainly not be ignored (since roughly 50% of the substance abusers in treatment in our program are also adult children of alcoholics). Similarly, if the person is currently living with a chemically addicted other, she would be referred to our family-members track—again with the knowledge that if this person enters our family program, ACOA issues will be attended to, since 60 to 70% of the other participants in these groups will also be ACOAs.

In a similar manner, when a family member comes for treatment because of problems coping with his spouse's addiction, a careful

---

*The offspring of alcoholics are at three to four times greater risk for developing alcoholism themselves than are the offspring of nonalcoholics (Bohman, Sigvardsson, & Cloninger, 1981; Goodwin, Schulsinger, Hermansen, Guze, & Winokur, 1973; Schuckit, Li, Cloninger, & Deitrich, 1985), and are also at greater risk for marrying substance-abusing partners (Black, 1981; Corder, McRee, & Rohrer, 1984; Gravitz & Bowden, 1984; Woititz, 1983).

alcohol and drug history is taken. If this family member has an alcohol problem, he is referred directly to our substance-abuse track.*

Making a Judgment Call: ACOA versus Substance-Abuse Group

The patient who presents for treatment around his ACOA issues but who is abstinent only a few months raises special issues regarding appropriate group placement. If the patient is solidly abstinent and no longer needs a place to focus on sobriety (or to be reminded that this is an issue for him), or if he has solid support elsewhere (e.g., in a 12-step program), it may be appropriate to consider the possibility of an ACOA group.† However, premature placement in a group that focuses on the ACOA issues may be used by the patient as a defense against examining his own substance abuse, concerns about drinking, or relapses, should they occur. Given that most substance-abuse groups will have a majority of members who are also adult children of alcoholics, and, given that any dynamically oriented group for substance abusers will explore family-of-origin issues, the more conservative placement, in most instances, is generally to put the patient in a dynamically oriented substance-abuse group. The goal is to avoid placing patients in a group where the group theme (e.g., ACOA group or family group) may make it harder for him to pay attention to more pressing issues that he needs to be attending to (e.g., his own substance abuse).

Assessing Alcohol and Drug Use

To facilitate the process of taking the initial alcohol and drug history, it is helpful to communicate to the patient that you are interested in the use of chemical substances and the patient's concerns about sub-

---

*It should be noted that the ACOA and relatives groups discussed in this chapter are intended specifically for non-substance-abusers. This is consistent with our view that ACOA and relatives groups should not be for currently active substance abusers or for patients still in early stages of recovery. The focus on parental or spouse abuse may not only distract from one's own focus on sobriety but may, at times, serve as a rationale for continued drinking.

†If the decision is made for placement in an ACOA group, it may be useful to have a contract with the patient that, should a lapse in abstinence occur, referral to a substance-abuse group instead, or in conjunction with, the ACOA group would be required.

stances (rather than focusing on substance *abuse*). Focusing on substance abuse is likely to increase resistance in those patients (family members or ACOAs) who are reluctant to connect any of their current problems with their *own* substance use—wishing to see the parent's or spouse's substance abuse as the primary source of current troubles. The alcoholic who may be abusing other drugs in addition to alcohol but who may not recognize this substance use as abusive may also be inclined to present a bland history if the emphasis is on *abuse*. It is thus important that a structured interview be carried out that actively enlists the patient in providing a detailed history of use of all mood-altering substances.

One of the more neutral ways of obtaining this information is to use an alcohol history questionnaire such as those included in Appendix C. (The first questionnaire is for those whose substance abuse is part of the initial presenting issue; the second is for patients who present initially around their ACOA issues.)

When a patient is asked about substance use, an important indicator that more exploration may be needed is the patient's categorical denial of any acquaintance with a given substance. For example, the patient may be asked, "Could you tell me something about your use of alcohol?" She responds, "I never drink." The therapist should then inquire, "How long has this been the case? Have you ever made an exception?" (and other similar explorations). In like manner, the patient should be asked, "Could you tell me something about your use of opiates—codeine, Percodan, morphine, etc.?" If the patient says, "I've never used any of these," the therapist should then inquire, "How about when you've had surgery, teeth pulled, bad coughs, headaches, etc.?" Unless specifically questioned, patients may give categorically negative responses in order to move the interview on and to avoid this area of inquiry. And unless further inquiry is actually carried out, it is difficult to assess whether a minimal response is due to resistance or genuinely reflects minimal usage. Patients may also assume—unless specifically asked—that any drug that has been *prescribed* does not count and is therefore not worth mentioning. The neutral questionnaire format will help the interviewer to cover the full territory in a way that feels relatively unthreatening to the patient (particularly if the focus is on a detailed overview of *use,* not abuse).

If you have gathered enough data to suggest the possibility of an alcohol problem, the Michigan Alcoholism Screening Test (MAST) (Hedlund & Vieweg, 1984; Selzer, 1971) may also be helpful. This questionnaire, which can be interviewer-or self-administered, includes 25 items covering social consequences of drinking, presence of addictive symptoms, interpersonal problems, and health problems associated with drinking. Items are differentially weighted, and the weighted item scores are summed. A total MAST score of 5 or above is indicative of alcoholism; a score of 4 is considered suggestive of problems with alcohol. The MAST has been more extensively used than any other alcoholism screening device and has been shown to be a sensitive, reliable, and valid measure (Selzer, Vinokur, & van Rooijen, 1975). Its only drawback is that it does not differentiate current from prior, but now resolved, alcohol-related problems. Accompanied by a good clinical interview, however, this differentiation should be relatively easy to make. (See Appendix D for a copy of the MAST and a scoring key.)

When taking an alcohol and drug history, it is important to encourage the patient to disclose as much information as possible. For example, if a patient is asked, "Can you tell me how much you have been drinking?" and she responds, "Generally three or four beers a night," I might ask, "When was the last time you recall having more than four?" I do not ask, "Do you ever have more than this?" but rather, "When did you . . . ?" assuming that a person who "generally" drinks three or four occasionally has more than this. My question contains the assumption that at times consumption will be greater and simply asks for more data. I might also ask, "What's the most you recall ever drinking in a single day?" and, "How long ago was that?" To stretch the limits of the patient's comfort in terms of discussing quantity of alcohol/drug use, when a patient says to me, "I'm not sure exactly how much I drink—a few drinks or so," I may start with some figures of my own—such as, "Is it more than a couple of pints a day?" I tend to start on the high end, because this indicates to the patient that I am used to figures like that, and it increases the perceived acceptability of any estimate that she may share.

In addition, when patients offer other kinds of vague responses, it is helpful to offer specifics that will help quantify their use. For example, a patient says, "I generally have two or three drinks a night." To this the interviewer should ask, "Do you measure your drinks? How big are they?" Or I might ask, "What size glass do you use." Or, if it is a mixed drink, "How many jiggers do you use in each drink?"

Relatively low frequency and quantity of drinking (for example, two or three drinks a couple of times a week) can often be in the "gray zone" in terms of our assessment of whether or not the person has a drinking problem. In such cases, information regarding quantity needs to be supplemented with information regarding the consequences of her drinking. The interviewer might ask, "Are you different after you have had two or three drinks?" "Does your husband ever think it's a problem?" or "Does anybody think that you should be drinking less?"

Assessing Patients in Terms of Quality of Abstinence

The group leader assessing potential new members for his substance-abuse group needs to assess: (1) where his group currently stands with regard to abstinence (as well as other crises in the group), (2) how the new member will fit in terms of the sturdiness of her commitment to abstinence and her general stability, and (3) whether the new member's entrance will be productive for the group. These are the same kinds of considerations one makes in any kind of long-term therapy group. Bringing in a new member who is in crisis may at times tax the group beyond its ability to function effectively. Yet, a person in similar crisis might be easily contained by the group at a different point in time—perhaps even adding a new dimension to the group.

A person in similar crisis might also be contained by the group if her emotional resources are reasonably solid. Thus, it is important to consider where a potential member stands in terms of her level of psychological functioning and integration, the kinds of defenses that she uses to maintain abstinence, and the rigidity of her defenses. Some recovering people 3 years into recovery are poorly integrated, crisis prone, and use relatively primitive defenses to maintain their abstinence—sloganism, and a rigid, dogmatic acceptance of AA principles. Such individuals want to "keep it simple," "avoid strong feelings," "live only in the present," etc. For these recovering people, the defenses that they use may, indeed, help them to stay abstinent. However, mixing such patients into a group with considerably more psychological sophistication has to be evaluated carefully. When new members are considered for placement in groups, how one maintains abstinence (the defenses and adaptations one uses) is as important as how long one is abstinent.

The extent to which AA is used as part of the adaptation to recovery needs special attention. Some groups develop a culture in which they expect all members to seriously embrace AA and to attend meetings regularly. In such a group, a member who is hostile or antagonistic to AA—even if he has maintained a long period of abstinence without it—may not be readily accepted by the group. In other groups, members may be less involved in AA. Any serious discrepancy along this dimension (assuming the leader decides the group can handle it) needs to be discussed during the pregroup interview in order to prepare the potential member for the fact that this may be an area of difference between him and the rest of the group.

The Pregroup Interview: Content and Format

Overview of Content

Pregroup interviews provide an opportunity for the group leader to supplement whatever information she has from the referring person about the patient, to further assess the patient's appropriateness for her group, to find out what the patient wants to work on, and to help shape his expectancies about what life in group will be about. I generally structure the pregroup interview(s) to cover the following topics: (1) what the patient is hoping for (the problems that he wishes to work on in the group, and his goals for treatment); (2) the treatment contract—how the group works and what will be expected of the patient (as well as what he, in turn, can expect from the leader and other group members); and (3) the patient's thoughts about resistances that are likely to emerge, that is, the ways that he characteristically avoids difficult or painful situations that are likely to be expressed during the course of his group work. Problems with the contract in the initial pregroup interview(s) may give clues to this, as well as how the patient handles the pregroup interview itself (e.g., failure to show up for the first scheduled meeting, lateness). Finally, (4) I ask the patient to share anything else that he feels would be helpful to know about him that is likely to influence his behavior in the group. This is an open-ended question and gives the patient an opportunity to share material that may not have been touched on but that may, indeed, be important to understanding the patient's dynamics and his subsequent interactions within the group.*

Generally speaking, I allow for two (often more) half-hour pre-

---

*I find this open-ended question helpful also in the beginning phase of individual therapy—after I have completed taking a more or less formal history.

group interviews. Although an argument can be made for a single longer interview, I believe that more data is available with regard to early resistance (lateness, no-shows, etc.) when the patient is given an opportunity to come back more than once. In addition, the patient has an opportunity between the first and subsequent interviews to think about the group guidelines as well as new anxieties that have been raised as the result of the initial pregroup interview(s), and then to explore these issues with the therapist before coming into the group. In my experience, more extensive contact with the therapist prior to actually entering the group often helps to "contain" more anxious patients who, as a result of the repeated contacts, will have a connection with at least one person (the therapist) upon entering the group.

Pregroup in the Same Room

The format that I particularly like for the initial encounter between a potential new member and the group involves interviewing the new member in the group room just prior to the time the group is scheduled to begin. As the new member leaves the room, the group members line up outside ready to enter. This provides an opportunity for group fantasies to be heightened prior to the new member's entry into the group (since a limited amount of data is available from seeing the new person). It also provides an opportunity for the new group member to get a feel for the group, since this format provides a safe "sneak preview" for the new member, who has an opportunity to see that the existing members look like "regular folks."

Setting the Group Contract

It is important that the patient understand, before joining the group, what he can expect as a member and what will be expected of him. In our clinic, during the pregroup interview(s), patients are given a handout by the group leader that briefly describes the way our dynamically oriented therapy groups work and states specific ground rules (see Appendix E). Patients are told that a special feature of this kind of therapy group is that it provides a mirror of other important groups to which people belong and, as such, provides a setting in which to examine patterns of behavior with both individuals and groups. They are also told that it provides a special setting in which new ways of relating can be tried out. The importance of intermember participation is emphasized as well as the therapist's role in facilitating this. Ground rules include: regular and timely attendance, payment for sessions missed without prior notice, timely payment of bills, and notification at least 3 weeks prior to terminating. Confidentiality is stressed, and members are told that they will be expected to talk about important issues in their lives that cause difficulty in relating to others or in living life fully, as well as about what is going on in the group itself, as a better way of understanding their own interpersonal dynamics. Finally, in order to keep the group energy as much as possible within the group, patients are encouraged to keep outside-of-group contact to a minimum and are asked to discuss with the group any "relevant" discussions that come up outside.

No matter how specific and detailed the initial treatment contract, even the most explicit ground rules will be understood differently by different members and at different points in the group's history. Although the group ground rules that we use have been reworked a number of times to minimize ambiguity, misinterpretations by group members still occur. It is thus important—both when preparing patients during the pregroup interviews and whenever the ground rules come up at later points in the life of the group—that the review of the ground rules takes place as a *process* and not merely as an itemization of a list.

Delineating the contract not only provides an opportunity to shape the patient's expectations regarding appropriate group behavior but also gives leaders an opportunity to assess whether a given patient will be able to adhere to the contract (and is thus appropriate for their group). Often this takes more than one pregroup interview—particularly if it is unclear whether the patient has understood or fully agreed to all the terms of the contract. For example, a patient whose job requires frequent overnight trips may indicate that he is not sure that he can make it to the group every week; or another may worry in the initial interview whether her husband can reliably make it home early enough to provide child care on group nights. In both instances, the leader, stressing the importance of regular and timely participation, might also explore whether another group that meets at a different hour or on a different night might increase the patient's ability to make a full commitment. The patient should then be encouraged to think about various possibilities, with the option of either requesting referral to a different group or meeting with the present leaders again to establish a firm commitment. Pregroup time (even if it takes several interviews) spent making sure that patients really understand the ground rules and are able to commit to them pays off in the long run in terms of maintaining stable groups. It also lays the groundwork for effective management of treatment issues throughout the life of a group.

The importance of the pregroup interview for shaping expectations and developing norms for effective group behavior is highlighted by a series of studies described by Frank (1985). He and his colleagues gave one group of patients (the experimental group) an initial role-induction interview that clarified the purpose of treatment and helped the patient behave in a way that was consistent with the therapists' image of a good patient. Compared to a control group of patients who were treated identically except that they lacked the preparatory interview, the experimental group (those receiving the role-induction interview) behaved more appropriately in therapy and had better outcomes.

Dealing with Simultaneous Membership in Other Groups

AA/Al-Anon and Group Therapy: It is common for substance abusers, family members, and ACOAs to be members of a 12-step program (e.g., AA, NA, Al-Anon) at the time they enter a therapy group. In fact, for many, membership in AA or Al-Anon may be the only kind of group treatment that they have experienced before joining a therapy group—an experience that is likely to have a strong influence on their expectations about group therapy.

It is thus important, after ascertaining that the patient is familiar with one of the 12-step programs, to underscore the ways in which the ground rules of therapy groups differ. Thus, for example, I might say to the patient, "Have you been using AA?" If the patient responds affirmatively, I might say, "Good, that can be a very helpful support, and we encourage it. However, it may be helpful for us to review some of the ways that participation in a therapy group differs a little bit from participation in AA." Then, as I review the ground rules with the patient, I might highlight the ways in which they differ from membership in AA—namely, that membership in a therapy group carries with it the expectation that patients will be at the group every week and on time, will call in if for some reason they are unable to come, and will give advance notice to the group should they consider discontinuing membership. It may be helpful to say to the new member, "In a therapy group you are expected to attend every week and on time; it makes a difference to people whether or not you are at a particular session. And, unlike AA, where if one needed to leave early one could, in the group it would matter a great deal to other members if somebody had to depart from the group prior to the end of the session." The boundaries are much tighter in a therapy group than in AA, there is more accountability, and people's comings and goings from the group are attended to more carefully.

Although these ground rules are not unique to therapy groups for substance abusers and their family members, and would be stated as part of the initial treatment contract for any therapy group, it is particularly important that they be underscored at the pregroup interviews with these populations because they do differ substantially from the ground rules of AA and Al-Anon.* Other ways in which the therapy group may differ from AA and Al-Anon should also be clarified. These include the expectation that members will pay, that outside-of-group contact has to be brought back into the group, and that what goes on in the group itself will be talked about (i.e., exploration of the group process itself). It may be especially important to attend to the latter, because most of the exchanges in large open groups in AA occur between the "leader" (i.e., the speaker) and various members. Most of the interaction is dyadic and not group interactional. Although this may be modified somewhat in smaller meetings or special step meetings, for many patients their experiences in 12-step programs will have exposed them to serial dyadic communication rather than group interaction among many members.

Finally, it is important to underscore that the group will focus on feelings and learning to communicate them more clearly, and will explore the past as well as the present with the goal of better integrating and understanding one's life experiences and feelings. Although patients will sometimes feel that there is conflict between their AA or Al-Anon experience and group therapy because the formats are so different, the therapist should be clear in his own mind that the two are not in any way mutually exclusive but, rather, serve different functions and provide support in distinct but complementary ways.

---

*I refer here to AA and Al-Anon for the sake of brevity but include, also, NA and Nar-Anon.

Education Task Group and Group Therapy: Not only are substance abusers and family members likely to be members of AA or Al-Anon while participating in a therapy group, but often they will also have had experience in a task-oriented substance-abuse education group. Like membership in AA or Al-Anon, participation in groups that have a substantial didactic component carries with it a prescribed set of expectations and ground rules that differ from the ground rules of a therapy group. It is thus helpful in the pregroup interview to prepare new members by differentiating group therapy not only from a self-help group but also from an education group. The therapist may say directly, "The purpose of this group is not so much to give you answers and provide information, but rather, to help you explore and better understand feelings and situations that you find difficult to manage, and to better understand where you fit in with the difficulties that you experience."

Anticipating Resistance

During the pregroup interview(s) it is also generally a good idea for the group leader to prepare the potential group member for the likelihood of resistance emerging at various points along the way—perhaps in the form of wishes not to attend on a given night, withdrawing from the group in silence, etc. Patients should be told that this is not uncommon and happens to most people at one point or another once they get into the work of therapy, but that what is most important is that the patient talk about these kinds of feelings rather than act on them. It is also helpful if, during the pregroup interview, leaders can anticipate with new group members the ways in which they are likely to resist or pull back that are familiar to them from other aspects of their lives. The therapist and patient may then agree that when these behaviors occur, they will serve as signals that something important is going on that needs to be talked about in the group.

Dealing with Anticipatory Anxiety

One important task of the pregroup interview(s) is to help patients process their fears about how their first night will go. Leaders can provide helpful assurance that all new members initially feel anxious and that this is quite to be expected. The patient may be asked, "What do you imagine other members have felt when they thought about the group before they first entered?" or "How do you think others would feel entering a new group?" Once members are actually in the group, it is also useful to have existing members talk about how it was for them in the beginning. The leaders might encourage this by asking "Do others of you remember what your first night in the group was like?"

Dealing with Patient's Anticipatory Fears of Falling Apart

Patients interviewing for groups where there is known to be a strong family-of-origin focus (for example, ACOA groups) may sometimes express concerns about getting overwhelmed and "falling apart" as they delve into material from the past. In the pregroup interview, the leader should anticipate with patients that these kinds of feelings may occur, without creating an expectation that the patient will regress. Thus, it may be helpful to suggest to patients that it is not unusual for people to have strong feelings and reactions and initially to worry about them, fearing that they are going to experience the feelings as if they were kids again—but of course they are not. I might say, "You are now an adult who will be experiencing some of the same kinds of feelings as when you were younger, but this time in a structured situation. There may be flickers of those old feelings coming up, and you may be scared when this happens because the last time you were in touch with these feelings you were just a kid and did not have a safe place to deal with all that was going on inside." Thus, we are saying two things to the patient: first, that it is expected and appropriate that he will experience some of these old feelings from the past, and also that we will be able to contain them because the patient is not a child any more, and the group will provide a safe context in which to help him with the feelings.

Differentiating Leader Behavior during the First Sessions and Later Sessions

Because the therapist may function somewhat differently early on— doing more to lower anxiety, provide support, and actively shape the norms of the group—it may also be helpful for the group leader to let members know in the pregroup interview something about her general role and also, if it is a new group, the ways that her role may be a bit different during the first few weeks. Thus, it may be helpful to say, "In my role as group leader, I will be acting as a facilitator to the group. The group will generally set its own agenda, talking about whatever comes up that seems relevant, and I will participate as I feel it is useful to facilitate the group process." If it is a new group, it is helpful to add, "In the first few weeks I will probably be a little more active than later on—helping the group to cover certain territory that I think will be important for us in getting to know one another. After that I will be inclined to be less active—leaving more of the work and most of the setting of the agenda up to the group members."*

It should be noted that in my individual work with patients I often do something very similar. I may say, after assessing the initial problem and ascertaining that it makes sense for the patient and me to embark on a treatment course together, "In the first few sessions I generally like to take a history and to find out more about how some of the current difficulties that you are having relate to some of the things that have gone on for you in the past. During the next few sessions— probably two or three—I will be a bit more active than I will be later on, asking more questions and structuring things a bit more so that we can somewhat systematically cover the territory. After that, I will be somewhat less active, and the sessions will be less structured. You will bring up whatever comes to mind or whatever makes sense to you to be talking about."

Special Patient Issues in the Pregroup Interview

The Patient Who Claims He Has No Problem

Frequently, the patient presents for treatment describing the only problem as one that exists outside of himself. Thus, such a patient may indicate that he is there "only because the court is requiring it"—that he was picked up for drunk driving or for possession of drugs and, "other than that, there is no problem." For many patients, not really believing there is a problem, or seeing it as primarily a problem in someone else's eyes, is an early defensive reaction. These patients, who openly protest about not having a problem, differ only in degree from many patients who wonder initially to what extent they are in treat-

---

*A change in roles that is also advocated by Friedman (1989) and supported by a body of research reviewed by Dies (1983).

ment for themselves and to what extent because somebody else thinks they have a problem.

However, when the patient's view of the problem suggests that he is likely to be an extremely difficult candidate for treatment, particularly in a group, it may be helpful to indicate to him that your program treats people who have *problems* with substance abuse; if he does not have such a problem (that is, if his only problem is that somebody else thinks he has one and is requiring him to come to treatment), then your program has nothing to offer him. It may be helpful to state, further, that your program does not simply help people to serve out court-mandated probation requirements—if that is all he has come for, perhaps he should look for another therapist or clinic who might be satisfied to have him merely attend sessions without being engaged in treatment. Thus, I might say to such a patient, "I treat patients who have problems with substance abuse. The requirement for membership in my group is not simply that you show up each week—even if that might be enough for the court; rather, I take people in my group only if they believe that they have a problem that the group may be able to productively tackle."

The patient might also be told that there are others in the group who, from time to time, may also question the seriousness of their substance-abuse problems and who may share some of his ambivalence about treatment—something that is important to talk about in the group. Basically, in your role as leader, it is important that you are able to satisfy yourself that you are bringing a viable therapy candidate into your group. If you are not sure that there is something you can offer the patient (other than satisfying the court), it may be necessary to schedule an appointment to meet again—after the patient has had some time to think about it—to see if there are some viable treatment goals that you and he can work on together.

The Patient Who May Not Be Appropriate for Group

Even in group-oriented clinics that have liberal criteria for acceptance into groups, groups with different levels of functioning, and a broad philosophical view that most patients will benefit from group, there will be some patients who may not be appropriate for any long-term group. Often we question a patient's appropriateness based on prior clinic experience with her—that is, some kind of initial short-term group experience where some difficult aspect of her behavior (verbal abusiveness to other patients, frequent interruptions, etc.) has been apparent. When confronted with such a patient in a pregroup interview, it is often helpful to talk directly about the ways in which her behavior in group has already been difficult and to question whether group treatment is the best choice for her. It is important that the patient understand that you have her interest as well as the group's to consider—that you do not want to put her in a situation that is not going to work out well for her and that the behavior that you have noted would most certainly put her at odds with the group, making it hard to have a positive therapeutic outcome. With some patients, if you think the behavior is potentially modifiable, you may also ask the patient whether she thinks that she could contain this particular behavior.

It is often helpful to begin such a discussion empathically by identifying the objectionable behavior as something the patient does when she is feeling especially vulnerable (this is probably true of most people's most objectionable behaviors). Thus, I might say, "In the short-term group, I had the feeling that when you were feeling very anxious and concerned about your own situation, it sometimes became almost impossible for you to track what was going on with other people in the group. Thus, in your sense of urgency about your own situation, at times it was clear that you weren't aware that another person was still talking." If the patient seems as if she is interested in pursuing the group even after this feedback has been given, I might say, "Perhaps we ought to meet a few times individually to see if we can figure out some ways that we might be able to understand more about this particular behavior, and also whether there are some checks we can put on it so that when you are doing it, we have some way of signaling you so that it won't get in the way of your own work and the work of the group."

I might also say, "If I bring you into the group, I want to bring you in in a way that makes sense; but given what I have already observed about some of your group behavior, if you continued to do that, I don't know that a long-term group would be so very useful for you. I think the group would be on your case a lot and that would make it hard for you to feel good about the experience." I might also suggest that there might be other options that might be more workable, at least at this point in the patient's life when she is feeling so very stressed. For example, it might make more sense for her to meet with her individual counselor weekly for a while and to reconsider the group option at a later point. An example will illustrate.

> *A young woman who seemed to be an "uncontainable interrupter" in her short-term therapy group wanted to continue in a long-term group. I had supervised her therapist's work in the short-term group and was thus familiar with her dynamics. In this instance, prior to referring her on to a long-term group, I decided, in my capacity as Clinic Director, that I would meet with her myself to explain my dilemma in making a long-term group referral. I laid out for her the problems that I understood she had been having in the short-term group—noting that when she seemed to be feeling a lot of stress, she would cut other people off, and wondered whether she felt there was something that she might be able to do about this behavior. I also suggested that for her to get what she needed from the group, she would need to be able to spend a lot more time listening and considerably less time talking in the group than she had been accustomed to. She indicated that she thought she could control both the interruptions and the amount that she spoke. She also indicated that she would be receptive to having the group members or the group leaders point out to her when her behavior was becoming disruptive and that, in the long run, this would be helpful to her. I asked her to think about it for a few days, and when we met a second time the patient was equally determined to try to monitor and work on this aspect of her behavior in the group. I agreed to refer her to a long-term group—with the understanding that she would discuss this with her new group leader in the pregroup interview, and if this disruptive behavior became unmanageable once she was in the group, we would consider an alternative treatment option. The patient joined her new group a few weeks later; and for the first 3 months in group she barely spoke at all unless addressed. With time her behavior in group became more spontaneous, and she remained in the group for 2 years.*

The Co-Led Pregroup Interview

If a group will have two leaders, the pregroup interview should be arranged, whenever possible, so that both co-leaders can be present. It is important for incoming members to have a sense not only of who both co-leaders are but also of how they interact with one another and what the combination is like. In those unusual circumstances where timing precludes the possibility of the two leaders doing the interview together, each one interviewing the patient individually is an alternative—although not nearly as desirable. In the pregroup interview, to avoid overwhelming the patient by a "two-on-one" approach (the two leaders both questioning the patient), it may help if the leaders talk to one another. This helps take some of the heat off the patient and also sets the tone for the kind of collegial interaction that will be occurring between the therapists. One of the leaders may start out, for example, reviewing the group ground rules and then may turn to the other and ask, "Are there any other ground rules that we've missed?" They may also consult with one another about what would be the best next step for the patient at this point. For example, one might say to the other, "You know, given the problems that Mr. Smith has in terms of some of the transportation issues that he has raised, I'm wondering if it might be useful for us to have a chance to meet with him again in a week and see whether any of the difficulties that he anticipates can be worked out. What do you think?" The leaders would then both have an opportunity to give each other feedback about how each views the situation, and the patient would be likely to feel less on the spot than if all the questions were directed to him.

Another part of the co-led pregroup assessment may take place as the group leaders check in with the patient about how he feels the interview is going—that is, whether any of the concerns he may have about the group experience, especially about interacting with two leaders, are being paralleled by the feelings that he is now having in the pregroup interview.

Minimizing Early Dropout

Group leaders are almost universally concerned about the stability of their groups and the problems raised when new members come in who are precariously connected to the group and who leave prematurely. If the goal is to get as many patients attached to a long-term therapy group as possible, the sooner the patient is attached to the continuing-care group following the intensive phase of treatment (be that the inpatient treatment phase, or an intensive day or evening program) the better. On the other hand, patients' initial motivation to continue treatment, often based on sudden panicky feelings about returning to the world that they left behind during the 2–4 weeks that they were in a structured program, may fade with time. Thus, the longer the delay and the greater the number of pre-group interviews, the more likely it is that only the more motivated patients will continue. The time delay and the pre-group interviews serve as another test of how motivated the patient will remain once she is out of the highly structured phase of treatment.

A middle ground between prompt placement of every patient (and dropout, soon after, of many of them) and delayed placement (which may lose patients who potentially could have been engaged had they been placed sooner) is to establish an intermediate group for patients to join as they are leaving the structured phase of treatment and for several weeks following (Vannicelli, 1988). This "transition group" might begin either prior to the end of the structured program or immediately after it has been completed and extend for a time-limited period, perhaps 5 or 6 weeks, after which referrals would be made to long-term groups. The option might also exist for patients to continue in this transition group for as long as they like in a "drop-in" capacity. This intermediate group thus serves as a continued support for all patients regardless of whether or not they are ready to make a commitment to a long-term weekly group, and also gives group leaders a chance to see how much of a commitment patients are actually ready to make. It thus provides the advantages of both delayed placement into a long-term group and a containing placement for patients during the peak stress period immediately following the intensive treatment phase.

Another step to minimize early dropout is to clearly articulate in the pregroup interview that it is very natural for patients to feel scared when they first enter a new group and worried about how it will all work out—that is, to get "cold feet." A new member's concerns about whether or not she has made the right decision are common at the beginning, and patients should be told this. They should also be told "part of the reason that we are talking about this with you now is that it's very important that you have a sense of what you are getting into; our group expects people who join to take it seriously and to really try to give it a shot." The leader might then say to the patient, "If you have any worries about whether if you get 'cold feet' you'll to be able to stay, maybe we need to talk again another time to give you a little more time to think about whether you are ready to make this kind of commitment."

I might also ask the patient how she typically handles it when she does get "cold feet," and if she would be willing to agree, even if she initially felt uncertain about whether she had made the right decision, that she would give it enough time (our clinic groups ask for at least 3 months) to see if, indeed, she could get comfortable in this group. With this kind of preparation, when the patient does get frightened and feels like bolting, the leader can remind her about the discussions that were held in the pregroup interview. Thus, the leader might comment, "This is just the kind of thing that we were talking about in the pregroup interview when we worried about the possibility that you might get scared early on; my hope is that you will stay with us at least long enough to understand more about why you feel that you have to leave so quick." The message should clearly be, "We are not closing the door so that you can't get out, but rather, would like you to see if you can stay and talk with us about it so that perhaps you won't feel that you have to leave."

This chapter has examined some of the structural issues that the group leader must consider in setting up a therapy group and procedures for selecting and preparing the members. Procedures were detailed for careful prescreening of members, including a detailed alcohol and drug history. Finally, considerable attention was given to the pregroup interview and its important role in shaping member expectations. The next chapter considers some of the issues that the leader must address when he actually assembles the members and begins the group.

❖ 4 ❖

Beginning the Group

Although the territory is mapped out in the pregroup interview, the journey actually begins with the first group session. The group leader's initial task is to help the group bond so that group members will feel safe in assuming a self-reflective pose while interacting with one another in the immediate present.

Maximizing the Opportunity for Visual and Verbal Contact

It is the therapist's responsibility to provide an appropriate environment for the group—one that is pleasant, relatively free of outside noise and distractions, and spatially arranged to allow for maximal intermember contact. The latter is too often not adequately attended to. It is most important that the room space be adequate to allow for a circle to be formed and, before the meeting, that leaders position chairs so that all members will have easy visual access to one another. Arrangements where some of the patients are side by side (for example, along a couch), where the chairs are of different heights, or where members' views of one another are obstructed by other pieces of furniture (lamps, tables, etc.) are less than ideal and should be avoided.

A group can get off to a shaky start when some members have difficulty making contact with one another visually and are too inhibited (as many members are, initially) to move their chairs in such a way as to regain contact. As a leader, if I find myself in such a situation—that is, where for some reason my view of a given patient is blocked, I actively squirm and noticeably move my chair back and forth, making as many adjustments as necessary. My behavior thus signals that I want to maximize my ability to see *everyone*.

In addition, for the first session it is helpful to set out the same number of chairs as members ultimately expected (i.e., the number who have been interviewed and who have agreed to participate) even if not all of them will be present the first session. This sets the stage so that members have some idea about what to expect in terms of group size.

Helping Members Begin

The leaders will want to help the group feel comfortable in the beginning and may be slightly more active the first session than later on—structuring introductions, sharing expectations, etc. The tasks that are important to cover the first night include the following: (1) introductions—each member should, at the very least, have an opportunity to say his name and *something* about himself; (2) sharing of goals—what each member is hoping to get out of being in the group; and (3) a review of the group contract.

I usually begin by asking group members if they know one another. I ask the question in this way not only because it provides an opportunity for people to do the introductions but also because it immediately opens up the issue of people who may know each other from another context. This is important because many of our patients have prior connections with one another (usually benign, through meetings that they attend or programs that they have participated in together—but sometimes not so benign), and it is important to uncover potentially difficult connections right at the outset.

Next, I will say to group members, "In the pregroup interview, each of you shared with me something about the goals that you had for your work in the therapy group. Perhaps it would be helpful to let other group members know something about what each of you are hoping to accomplish here." If during the first two tasks—introductions and sharing of individual goals—the group gets bogged down and one or two members take up too much of the time, I would say to the group, "I think it's real important that other members also have a chance to get to know one another tonight; perhaps we could take another 10 minutes to hear something about each of the rest of you."

It is important in the first session that every member get a chance to speak.

Finally, the group ground rules will be discussed. I might begin by saying, "Each of you had a chance during the pregroup interview to review the group ground rules, and I wonder if any thoughts or questions about those ground rules have come up for any of you since then." I would then ask members what they remember about the ground rules, letting group members spontaneously recall as many as they can. I would reward appropriate responses by saying, "Yes, that's an important one," and would modify any that come up in a distorted fashion by asking others in the group what they recall about that particular ground rule. I would also call special attention to any ground rules that get omitted, possibly just noting that it is *interesting* that a given rule was omitted, possibly exploring whether there might be something about this *particular* ground rule that was especially hard for people—at least to remember. (In my private groups, the ground rule that is most frequently forgotten is the unpopular one about having to pay for every session regardless of whether members are present or not.) After the discussion of the ground rules I might pass out a written copy, once again, for members to take home.

It is particularly important that within the first few sessions all members feel that they have a place in the group. Thus, if the leader notices that one member has not participated very much in any of the early sessions, it may be helpful to comment, "We haven't heard much from you tonight, Jane, but perhaps next week the group will have a chance to get to know you a little bit more." We want to be sure that no member walks away feeling totally ignored or feeling that her presence has not been noted.

Since it is hoped that all group members will begin to feel connected to the group early on, specific interventions may be useful for promoting group cohesion. Alpert (1990)* suggests several strategies for this. Pointing out that it is important for each group member to make a connection with at least one other member, she suggests that this kind of bonding can be facilitated by the leader's active efforts to "make links whenever possible" between members—for example, by underscoring similarities. Thus, the leaders may say, "It seems that Sue

---

*Geraldine Alpert. "The Rapid Turnover Group." Workshop presented at the Annual Meeting of the American Group Psychotherapy Association, Boston (1990).

and Bob, and perhaps others in here as well, are struggling with very similar problems with their anger." Occasionally, particularly in the initial sessions, group members may present what appears to be a united front *against* perceiving themselves to be similar to one another—each claiming, for example, how "unique and different" his situation is. Even here, a sense of commonality can be created by the leader, who may comment, "This sense of being different in some important way is something that you all have in common."

Other strategies that may be helpful, initially, in building cohesion are also described by Alpert: (1) encouraging thoughts about the group between sessions, for example, by asking members to share thoughts that they have had about the group as a whole or about individual members during the week that has intervened since the last meeting; and (2) "underlining subtle positive feelings about the group that are not yet fully apparent"—a technique that Alpert refers to as "pump priming for positive group feeling." The group leader can prime the pump in this way by turning a chorus of complaints about "how hard it was to get here tonight" into a statement of the group's emerging value for its members. Thus, the leader may say, "It has taken some real effort for each of you to get here tonight, yet each of you has made a point of doing so—an indication, perhaps, of some of the hopeful feelings that are beginning to develop."

In the first few meetings there also may be more need for "greasing of the wheels" by the group leader. Since some members will be embarking on their first group therapy experience (or perhaps their first therapy experience), it is to be expected that some will have "cold feet." A number of strategies may be useful in helping members to deal with initial awkwardness and hesitancy about how to proceed. For example, when group silences occur, leaders may intervene more directly by asking, "What makes it hard to begin?" or, "What makes it hard for the group to continue?" In addition, individual patients who are silent during much of the initial session may need special attention. Leaders may draw in such members initially by commenting, "Some people seem to be finding it difficult to enter," and wondering, "What may make it difficult?"

Greasing the wheel may also take the form of supporting positive group behavior, thereby helping to establish norms for effective group participation. For example, to the hesitant patient who says, "I'm really not sure what's supposed to happen here—I'm kind of uncertain about where to begin," the leader might respond, "What you're doing right now is just what we're hoping for in here—you are sharing with us in an open, straightforward manner exactly what you're feeling just as it comes up." We are thus telling the hesitant patient that he is on the right track and that his earnest self-disclosure (reflected in his faltering comment) is just what is needed for the group to be able to begin (Alpert, 1988). The leader might say, "Joe, what you're doing right now is just what needs to happen in a group like this. You are sharing some of your feelings in the present moment about what it's like to be here and your uncertainty about the whole thing." Thus, the patient is being told that he does know what to do and is, in fact, doing it.

Other supportive remarks may also be helpful that will communicate that it is natural not to know quite how this enterprise is going to work out in the beginning. Thus, I might also say something like, "My guess is that a lot of you aren't quite sure yet just what is going to happen here; its going to take some time to know what this venture is all about"; or, "My guess is that many of you—perhaps most—are feeling a little bit anxious tonight, and that's pretty natural considering that we are embarking on something that's a little bit unknown to each of you." Basically, my stance is to be a bit more supportive and a bit more active than I may be in later sessions.

Leader comments that may also be helpful in the beginning are those which help members to establish norms of interacting with one another. Thus, the leader might comment, "I wonder how others are responding to what Jane has been sharing," or might notice body language that indicates responses that have not yet been verbalized, with comments such as, "You seem to be responding to what Jane was sharing. Can you tell us something about what was going on for you as she was talking?"

While being initially more supportive and active, the leader must take care to avoid an interactive style that positions him as the center of a star in which all members end up communicating primarily with him. The facilitative remarks should be made only if they are needed to lower the level of anxiety in the group or to foster an initial sense of connectedness. The leader should *not* be more active than necessary and certainly should avoid inserting himself when interactions are spontaneously occurring among group members unless it seems important to change course. (Strategies for intervening, when this is indicated, are detailed further in the chapters that follow.)

Providing Appropriate "Boundaries" around the Group Time

Whenever possible, it is preferable if the leaders can be present both to "open" and to "close" the group. Thus, ideally, leaders will already be in the room and will have had an opportunity to arrange the chairs (and, when co-leading, to confer with one another) prior to the group's beginning. Keeping the group room door closed until the time the group begins and then opening it promptly at the starting time provides an even cleaner boundary, since patients do not then trickle in and begin small talk with one another or with the leaders prior to the official beginning of the group. Less desirable, though sometimes unavoidable, is the situation in which the group-room door is simply left open and members enter as they arrive, the leader joining them at the designated starting time. Although the leader's arrival thus signals the beginning of the group, this model has the disadvantage that the leader often feels that he has "interrupted something" that is already taking place.

Tidy boundaries around closing the group are equally important. Ideally, leaders will remain in the group room until the last member exits. When leaders must hasten to get away, leaving members to remain in the group room, the boundaries are less clear. (I have been told that some groups continue, without their leaders, for prolonged sessions after the close of the official group.) Although it may be true that group members do something somewhat similar in the lobby when they all exit together, the clear boundary around the official group space provides a safer, cleaner containing environment.

If a group is already in place in which boundaries are less clear-cut than the leader would prefer, remediation may be possible even if the group has been in existence for some time. For example, in one of our clinic groups in which leaders had other obligations just prior to the group, they had developed the habit of setting up the group room in advance and then going off to their other responsibilities on the hospital campus. They would then return just before the group was scheduled to begin but often felt, upon their arrival, that they were interrupting something that was already in process. They decided to modify this situation by telling group members that in the future the room would be kept locked until the leaders arrived, and members should wait in the waiting room until the group's designated starting time. In another group, where leaders needed to leave promptly at the end of the group but the group members often lingered on for lengthy postgroup sessions, the leaders similarly informed the group that in the future they would need to lock up the group room upon their departure. Thus, when the group ended, leaders stood at the door, keys in hand, until the last member exited.

Clear boundaries around the time frame of the group are also important with regard to members' arrivals and departures. A clear message should be given that members are expected to arrive on time and to remain for the entire session. There should be a clearly stated expectation that, regardless of how heated the group process may get, group members will remain in the room and talk about their feelings.

Maintaining the Boundaries of the Group: Intermember Interactions

The boundaries of the group will also be strengthened by clearly articulating the following ground rules: members are expected to attend regularly, to hold confidential what other members share, and to minimize outside-of-group contact. With regard to the latter, it is important that members have a shared understanding that although it is likely that members may see one another at AA or Al-Anon meetings, it is desirable to keep as much of the group energy as possible within the group. As Rutan and Stone (1984) indicate,

> The fundamental use of the group is for therapeutic, not social, purposes, and in the long run the two are mutually exclusive. (Thus) . . . it is more therapeutically profitable to discourage extra-group socializing, since doing so reduces the variables affecting group behavior and increases the likelihood of spontaneous revelation of affects in the group. (p. 110)

Thus, patients should be encouraged to keep outside-of-group contact to a minimum, and also to discuss with the group any "relevant" content that comes up outside. Although the word "relevant" is somewhat vague, and different members will surely interpret it in different ways, there should be a shared understanding that if the outside-of-group contact exceeds the usual socializing in the waiting room or at AA or Al-Anon meetings, it should be discussed with the group. It is sometimes helpful to give concrete examples—for instance, if two group members find themselves socializing extensively or having a "special" liaison; or if two group members find themselves discussing, even briefly, their feelings about other members, the leader, or the group itself. Discussion of these examples should help clarify that important relationships that take place outside and are not discussed with the group rob the group as a whole of the opportunity to explore these matters and rob the individuals involved of the opportunity to get valuable feedback from other members. Equally important, the outside-of-group business that does not get talked about within the group takes on the character of "special secrets," the existence of which runs counter to the group's shared goal of mutual openness and trust.

In the initial phases of the group, and also at times of stress in the group, members may move toward deliberately increasing the "social" aspect of the group. Although members may feel that this may help them to feel "closer" to one another, it also generally serves to dilute the intensity of the group work by creating a "safe" friendship network. Thus, group members may openly discuss in the group the possibility of social gatherings at one another's homes, postgroup pizza get-togethers, etc. Although our clinic group ground rules do not forbid this activity, our group leaders use a number of strategies to help shape the norms about minimal outside-of-group contact. First, when actual socializing or the wish to socialize comes up, leaders take an actively exploratory attitude about it, asking, "What does it mean to group members to have these socializing opportunities?" "How do members imagine that the group might be different were the socializing *not* to take place?" "What functions do members imagine that the socializing might serve for the group itself?" Leaders may also create an expectation that, once the group is fully under way and functioning at its highest potential as a therapy group, the socializing or the wish for socializing will decrease. Leaders might say something such as, "At this point, there seems to be a feeling that members cannot get enough from one another during our 1½-hour weekly meetings and that for members' needs to be adequately met, more time, different formats, etc. are needed. I have a hunch, however, that as we get to know one another better and really get down to the work that group members came for, the outside-of-group contact will decrease."

Shaping Group Norms with Forecasts and Hunches

At times, particularly early in the history of the group, it may be useful for the leader to make deliberate efforts to shape group norms concerning effective behavior that will promote the work of the group. One of my favorite shaping strategies (briefly illustrated in the previous section) is to make use of positive forecasts or "hunches." For example, to a group member who is reluctant to talk about a particularly painful area, the group leader might say, "I have a hunch that this is something you will feel more comfortable talking about as you know people in here better." Or, the therapist may "predict" a change in group behavior based on her knowledge of the way that groups develop. For example, in response to group members' outside-of-group contacts, the leader might comment, "In groups such as ours, outside-of-group contact generally diminishes as group members feel more comfortable with one another and more ready to begin to know one another in a different, more therapeutic kind of way." Group leaders may also encourage group members' willingness to discuss transference feelings with forecasts such as, "I'd expect that as we work together, members will come to have a variety of feelings about other members, as well as about the leaders, and will find it helpful to talk about these feelings."

Negative behaviors, too, can be commented on and "shaped" by the use of positive forecasts. For example, to the patient who repeatedly protests in any heated situation that she "has no feelings," a leader might posit, "I have a hunch that you, like all of us in here, have many different kinds of feelings and that, with time, we will come to understand more about them." Or, to the patient who rambles on and on with extensive details, the leader might predict, "I have a hunch that as you feel more understood in here, you will feel less pressured to provide us with quite so much detail when you explain what is going on for you." Many behaviors related to ground rules can similarly be "shaped" by forecasting positive performance in the future. For example, regarding lateness and absenteeism, a leader might comment, "I have a hunch that as members come to know that they can count on others to be here for them, greater efforts will be made to make this the very highest priority on Tuesday nights."

Basically, positive forecasts underscore that as group members come to have more positive feelings about the group (more trust, greater comfort, etc.) and that as the group gets down to work, certain kinds of positive or proactive behaviors are more likely to occur, and behaviors that get in the way of group growth will decrease. Such leader comments are useful, not only because they promote positive expectations and an aura of optimism, but also because they provide explicit guideposts that help the group and individual members to judge when progress is being made.

This chapter has examined several ways in which the leader sets the stage for the group members to bond and begin working together. The leader accomplishes this by providing an appropriate setting for the group, helping members to get started, providing adequate boundaries around the group, and by helping to shape norms that will promote the growth of the group. The next chapter examines special issues related to group growth and development that arise in groups for substance abusers, groups for ACOAs, and groups for other family members.

❖ 5 ❖
Special Population Issues

This chapter highlights issues and themes that are likely to assume particular importance in groups for substance abusers, in groups for collaterals of substance abusers (family members), in couples groups where one or both spouses are recovering, and in ACOA groups. While none of the issues discussed is totally unique to these populations, what differentiates these issues is their frequency of occurrence in the subgroups for which they are described and the importance of appropriate management, given their centrality to the ongoing group themes. Before discussing these special issues and themes, it is important to emphasize that the group work we do with each of these subgroups is, for the most part, very similar to the work we do with other generic psychiatric outpatient populations. This is consistent with our view of substance abusers, collaterals, and ACOAs as diagnostically heterogeneous groups of patients who vary considerably in terms of symptoms, presenting issues, and level of functioning. What differentiates our work with each of these subgroups is our focus on particular resistances (or roadblocks) that are characteristic of each population—for substance abusers, resistance to giving up alcohol and drugs (and other recovery-related defenses); for ACOAs and other family members, resistance to giving up the focus on the substance abuser.

In substance-abuse groups, specific issues that require careful consideration and preparation include (1) the patient's contract with the group regarding abstinence and the supports needed to maintain it; (2) management of substance-abuse episodes; (3) the need for active outreach to provide early intervention with patients who have missed a group session and may be abusing alcohol or drugs; (4) special confidentiality issues related to the frequency of communication in groups with substance abusers between the leaders and outsiders (other staff, family members, other patients, employers); (5) the group's defensive focus on drinking and drugging; (6) recovery-related defenses; and (7) vulnerability around holidays.

In couples groups when one or both members are recovering, special issues include: (1) communication problems within each couple, (2) the disequilibrium associated with recovery, (3) differentiating the couples group from Al-Anon; (4) learning to express anger appropriately, and (5) the special advantages of a male/female co-therapy team.

In groups for collaterals, special issues include: (1) disowning any problems in the self, (2) entrenchment in the quagmire of despair, (3) talking only about the significant other, and (4) the emergence of an alcohol or drug problem within a group member.

In groups for ACOAs, special issues include: (1) intense "family dynamics" and heightened family transference, (2) flight from the group (the wish to leave prematurely), (3) finding the identified family problem, (4) the search for a rescuer, (5) rigid role assignments, (6) hanging on, (7) negative self-view to preserve parental "goodness," (8) the ACOA label, (9) resistance to "taking a look" at what's going on, (10) concerns about predictability of authority figures, and (11) concerns about early problem drinking.

I discuss each of these special population issues as they arise within the context of long-term interactional therapy groups—providing specific techniques for addressing each issue.

GROUPS FOR SUBSTANCE ABUSERS

The dynamic interactional group therapy techniques that we use for outpatient substance abusers differ from those used with other outpatient populations in terms of the leader's active interventions in support of abstinence and explicit endorsement of the simultaneous use of other supports that will be helpful in maintaining it (including AA/NA, Antabuse, naltrexone,* etc.). We believe that abstinence is essential to the patient's eventual emotional stability, and stress this in

---

*Antabuse and naltrexone are prescribed substances, the former causing extreme dysthymia if combined with alcohol and the latter blocking the "high" associated with opiate ingestion.

the pregroup interview(s). However, group membership is not specifically contingent on abstinence, but rather, on the patient's willingness to struggle honestly about using alcohol or drugs (or the wish to use), with commitment to abstinence as a goal.

The Contract Regarding Abstinence

The group norm regarding abstinence should be made explicit as part of the initial group contract and should indicate that all members will be working toward abstinence, and that any difficulties encountered in working toward this goal (in the form of either fears about substance use or actual use) will be discussed with the group. The importance of a set of shared norms about what it means to be working on one's substance-abuse problem (as discussed in Chapter 3) cannot be underestimated. Thus, it is essential that the group leader, when preparing members for entry into the group, make it clear what the expectations are and that members will endorse an abstinence goal.

It is also important for the group leader to be prepared to set limits should lapses in abstinence occur—reminding the wavering patient about the shared group norm and the necessity of adhering to the group contract in order to continue membership. As discussed in more detail in the material that follows, it is the leader's job either to remind the wavering patient directly of the group ground rules or, when possible, to solicit this from other group members.* The decision about what to do when a patient fails to respect the group contract will have the most therapeutic benefit for the patient and the other group members if each is asked to give his own recommendation. A well-functioning group will be able to state its expectations and will set appropriate subgoals (e.g., the patient must start attending additional AA/NA meetings, must get a sponsor) with a clear time for resuming abstinence. In other words, there will be a clear focus on increasing the structure and supports necessary for maintaining the abstinence required for staying in the group.

At times the group may be too lenient (for example, when a member's substance use serves a function for the group or when others

---

*Much of this material and the material through page is elaborated in earlier papers (Vannicelli, 1982; 1987; 1988, Vannicelli, Canning & Griefen, 1984; Vannicelli, Dillavou & Caplan, 1988).

in the group are feeling anxious about their own potential drinking slips and are fearful that a stiff policy may mean that they too will be asked to leave). If such group reluctance persists, the leader will have to help the group understand its resistance to enforcing the contract and, at the same time, set the limits clearly herself.

Clearly, for the well-prepared leader, who is able to set limits appropriately and to negotiate adding the supports necessary for resuming abstinence, a patient's brief resumption of substance use should not necessarily lead to dismissal from the group. In groups with substance abusers, lapses from abstinence will certainly occur, since the course of recovery for many patients is punctuated with periodic setbacks. It is helpful for the therapist to view the recovery process favorably if the patient substantially increases the duration of abstinence and decreases the number and severity of substance-abuse episodes. A slip should not suggest to either the patient or the therapist that all that had been gained has now been lost. As Washton (1989) points out, "A slip must be addressed as an avoidable mistake, not as a tragic failure" (p. 109). In fact, a "slip" handled appropriately by the patient (i.e., the patient solicits help or stops using alcohol or drugs soon after the onset of the episode and discusses it openly with the group) can be a useful learning experience for the patient as well as other group members—underscoring the need for constant vigilance and adequate support for maintaining abstinence.

While it is clear that the well-prepared leader will never be laissez-faire about slips, neither will she give up good clinical judgment about how to proceed. Clarity, fast action and good clinical judgment are called for. In this regard, I lean towards a flexible attitude regarding whether or not a member can participate in the group the same day in which substance use has occurred. Clearly, the group is not effective either for the member himself or for the group as a whole if a member comes who is visibly intoxicated. However, the precise definition of intoxication is not an easy one, and there is a lot of territory between a noticeably intoxicated patient whose behavior is not appropriate for group (discussed in a later section) and a member who, perhaps a few hours before, has had a relatively contained slip (perhaps one beer).

Rather than having a rigid rule that members cannot participate if they have used *any* chemical substances within 24 hours of the group (a rule which I think often leads to withholding information about slips), I prefer a rule that clearly states that patients must be in an appropriate condition to participate in order to be at the group. This allows the therapist to make a clinical judgment, on a case-by-case basis, as to whether or not a patient who has slipped may benefit from being in the group that night. It is important that the therapist reserve the right to examine the status of the patient and to determine whether participation in the group will be clinically useful to that member (and others) if he comes to the session.

Let us take, for example, a patient who calls me a few hours before the group indicating that he "got really scared" earlier in the day, after taking a couple of sips of beer and pouring the rest down the sink. I would want to use my clinical judgment to decide whether it might be most helpful for the patient to come in and have a chance to review with the group: (1) what was going on that got him so close to being in serious trouble again, (2) how it was that he did not use his supports sooner, and also (3) what supports and strengths he did use in order to stop himself before things got more out of hand. The member who talks about a slip and being appropriately frightened by it can serve a useful role for the group. On the other hand, if a patient called me and said that he had been drinking heavily "a couple days ago" but sounded to me as if he might be intoxicated, I would suggest that perhaps he and I needed to get together prior to the group to find out more about what was going on for him. This would allow me to gather more information about whether or not the group would be useful for him that night.

Contracting for Increased Supports: Making It Realistic

While it is extremely important that the patient come into the group and talk about slips, it is also important that a philosophy be adopted by the group and reinforced by the leader's behavior, as well, that if a slip does occur—and in particular, if the slip becomes a "slide"*— that the member must embrace other supports in order to remain in the group. Thus, the therapist's position should be that slips are an indication that the current support system is not adequate to sustain the patient's solid commitment to abstinence and that the system of supports needs to be shored up. (This might involve increasing the number of AA or NA meetings, getting a sponsor, adding a relapse

---

*Marlatt's (1985) terminology is equally appropriate here in his discussion of "lapses" versus "relapses."

prevention group or an individual therapist to work on RP with her, adding Antabuse or naltrexone.) In our clinic this kind of contracting is part of the initial phase of treatment (during the individual assessment and contracting phase) even before patients participate in short-term 5-week groups, and is a familiar part of the treatment process by the time patients join long-term groups.

It is important, both in articulating the initial treatment contract and throughout treatment whenever a new contract has to be initiated or the old one updated, that the patient be actively and *realistically* engaged in the contracting process. It is our experience that a tough, unilateral contract that is "laid down" by the therapist is clinically effective only in those rare instances in which patients are in medical danger, such that any time lost between a drinking slip and getting them into treatment would seriously jeopardize their health. Such patients are told at the outset that should they have even a single drinking slip during the course of their evaluation, further treatment in our program would only be possible in the inpatient setting.

Except for these extreme cases, we are not in favor of tough, unilateral contracts imposed by the therapist early in treatment without sensitivity to the state of the treatment alliance. Such contracts, for the most part, will be effective only in keeping less motivated patients out of treatment. To cite an extreme example, a colleague from another program once stated, "I've never had anybody who drinks in any of my groups." When asked how he managed to do this, he replied, "Easy. Patients know that if they slip even once, I will kick them out." Indeed, this might have prevented some slips. But any patients who did slip were banished from treatment.

Less extreme but not uncommon, particularly with less experienced staff, are contracts that are made too early and that are too stiff for the patient to endorse. While the patient may give lip service to agreeing to the contract, when a slip or lapse does occur, the patient simply drops treatment rather than complying with the contract. For example, a recently abstinent patient might be told during the first outpatient interview that if she has a drinking slip before the next session, she will have to begin Antabuse and attend six AA meetings per week. She may agree to this during the first hour. It may not even occur to her at this point that she is still in serious jeopardy for the possibility of drinking. However, should a slip actually occur at this point, it is not likely that she would follow through on such stiff terms. It would be more likely that she would drop treatment instead.

A carefully negotiated contract requires that the patient be actively engaged in the process; this also requires that a treatment alliance be established. A carefully negotiated contract will be sensitive to the current status of the patient's alliance and will offer gradations of increasing support that the patient is actively involved in selecting and can readily endorse (see Griefen, Vannicelli, & Canning, 1985, for a detailed case example). This means that the therapist and patient together must decide what would be an effective and workable plan. "Ready-made" solutions proposed by the patient such as "90 meetings in 90 days," or "60 meetings in 60 days" should be carefully challenged. For example, when a patient says, "I'll just do 90 in 90", the therapist should inquire, "Is that realistic for you? How have you done with those kinds of commitments in the past? Given the many other things that you have in your life right now, will you be able to do that?" The patient should be encouraged to embrace a plan that she really can do. A more modest plan that she can reliably carry out is more likely to succeed than an ambitious plan that is verbally endorsed but not likely to be followed, leading to discouragement and a sense of failure. I might inquire further, "How many meetings are you sure you can do?" I might even encourage a patient to start with a more modest plan, see how that works out, and, after a few weeks, decide what changes might be in order.

Dealing with Specific Drinking/Drugging Hurdles

So far we have been talking about appropriately handled slips. However, there is a lot of ground between an appropriately handled slip and other forms of drinking and drug use that occur within the context of the group therapy. Four of the most common drinking and drugging landmarks (from least to most common) are the following: (1) coming to the group visibly under the influence and unable to interact appropriately with other group members; (2) drinking or using drugs between sessions but refusing to acknowledge it, even when directly confronted by group leaders and members; (3) use of substances which is talked about but in which there is no intention of stopping; and (4) periodic substance abuse that is appropriately discussed and during which the patient continues to verbally endorse the group norm of abstinence—while his behavior contradicts it.

Coming to the Group Intoxicated

The patient who comes to the group intoxicated not only defies the group norm but frequently, if allowed to remain, makes it impossible for the group to proceed. If it is immediately obvious to the group leaders that a member is unable to participate because of intoxication, the member should be asked to leave and to return in a condition appropriate for participation the next week.* More difficult is the patient whose intoxication is not immediately apparent but who becomes disruptive during the course of the meeting. It should be explained to the patient that his specific alcohol- or drug-related behaviors—e.g., talking while others are talking, inability to keep up with what is going on in the group, inability to sit still—indicate that he is not able to participate reasonably in the group that evening. Ideally, in such an instance the patient would simply get up and walk out and let the group go on. But intoxicated patients are rarely so accommodating. It is often helpful if the leader couples his observation that the patient is having difficulty participating with a suggestion that he go out and get a cup of coffee or some fresh air and return only when he feels that he can participate appropriately. (This is somewhat less rejecting than simply asking a patient to leave, and less likely to evoke a struggle. Thus, compliance is more likely—a particularly important consideration once the session has already begun.

Whether or not the patient returns that evening, the group members should be encouraged to share their feelings and observations about both the patient's behavior and the therapist's request that he leave. (Group leaders should be prepared for possible anger from group members who may see the leader's "invitation" to the patient to leave as punitive or rejecting, and they should be prepared to discuss this with the group.) When the patient returns the next week, group members should be asked to share their feelings with him about what happened the previous week, and he and the group should be asked to discuss what is to be done (as indicated above).

A special variation of the problem of an intoxicated member occurs when it is apparent that *someone* in the group has been drinking

---

*Provision must also be made for assuring the patient's safety if he is not in condition to get himself safely home. A check-in with the patient prior to the next group session is also generally indicated—at least by telephone and preferably in a face-to-face meeting with the leaders.

(because there is a distinct odor of alcohol in the room) but the leader is uncertain who it might be. Even if the therapist has no idea who it is that might be drinking, it is essential that he not ignore the smell of alcohol in the room. One way of dealing with this is for the therapist to inquire, "I wonder if what is going on in here right now might relate in some way to the faint odor of alcohol in the room?" (Thus, the presence of the odor is presented as a fact.) Or, the leader may simply state, "There is a faint smell in here that seems like it could be alcohol"—again inquiring about the thoughts and feelings that people have about this.

Often the leader is tempted to say something like, "I smell alcohol; does anyone else?" This is generally less effective, as it opens the possibility for a debate about whether or not there is a smell, rather than directing the group to the fact and then letting them discuss the feelings that go with it. The problem with this kind of "leading the witness" inquiry, in which the leader asks the group for support, is that whether or not members go along may depend as much on whether they feel like supporting the leader as it does on their belief in his accuracy. And a group that is angry at the leader (as well it may be if a member is doing poorly) might be inclined to withhold support, as a show of outrage. Thus, a more direct approach on the part of the leader is called for. Even if it is not immediately apparent who in the room may be drinking, the issue has not been ignored, and with time, clarity is likely to emerge.

"Using" but Refusing to Acknowledge It

Since most substance-abuse treatment groups exist within the context of a larger treatment system, it is not uncommon to learn from sources outside the group (other staff, patients, a concerned spouse, an employer) that a patient is using alcohol or drugs but is not talking about it in the group. When the therapist obtains information of this sort, he should use it to help the patient talk about what is going on. (It should be clear, again from the initial contract, that there will be no secrets, and certainly that any information that the therapist receives will be shared with the patient.) Ideally, the therapist will use the information to help the patient disclose her substance use "on her own." This can be facilitated by starting out with a general comment such as "I understand, Sandy, that you've been having rather a tough time for the past several weeks." If the patient acknowledges this, she is then asked to share as much about it as she can with the group. If she does not mention her use of alcohol or drugs, or if she denies that there have been any problems, the therapist should share in a factual way whatever information he has received. (For example, "Your husband called in this evening and was concerned that you might be drinking"; or "Your counselor, Mr. D, tells me that he ran into you in the subway where you were quite visibly high.") If denial persists, the patient should be asked what sense she makes of the discrepancy between the outside information and her own report.

If it is clear that the patient is not able to trust the group enough to talk about her substance use, this dilemma should be presented to the patient: "It must be hard for you, Sandy, to find yourself in a group in which you don't feel safe enough to talk about your drinking." (It is sometimes helpful at this point for the group as a whole to explore feelings of safety in the group and each member's sense of what she feels she can and cannot share.) In any case, the patient must be reminded of the group contract regarding working toward abstinence and talking about slips if they do occur, and she should be asked to decide whether she can work within this group norm. If there is an indication that the substance abuse continues and still is not discussed, the therapist will have to let the patient know (preferably in the group) that, at this point, she and the group have an unworkable relationship, and she should be asked to leave.

Another difficult situation for the leader to handle is a patient who comes in showing signs of intoxication (perhaps a faint smell, disheveled appearance, slightly slurred speech, etc.) who, when confronted, denies that he has been using substances. To this individual it might be appropriate to say something such as, "Bill, you seem somewhat less tidy about your appearance this week than usual, and I am also smelling alcohol in the room. I'm concerned that you may be drinking." I might then ask the group if other members have also been concerned about Bill. Even if the group does not support this, and even if Bill denies that he has been drinking, I might further comment, "My hunch is, Bill, that it's been difficult for you to acknowledge that you've been having a hard time with alcohol because you care so very much about what people in here think of you and you're afraid of disappointing them." This is an empathic response that says to the patient, I can understand your not leveling with us—it's not that you are a bad person or that you want to put one over on the group, but rather that you are worried about what people will think of you. In my own experience, I have found that patients are sometimes willing to assent to an empathic comment such as this even when direct questions about whether they have been drinking continue to be refuted.

Occasionally group members may confront Bill following such an intervention by saying, "Oh, so you have been drinking!" If Bill again says, "No," it would be helpful for the group leader to ask the group what they had just heard Bill say (in the prior intervention) and why it seems so important to have him "make a confession." If Bill gives a positive response to my empathic statement about his drinking and about his difficulty talking about it, I would simply move on to ask the group to process what they think needs to happen next in order to help Bill get "squared away" again—the time frame for the resumption of abstinence, additional supports that need to be added and, possibly, some way of establishing a safer forum with Bill so that he will be able to talk about the drinking if it does happen again.

At times such as this, the possibility of urine screens may also be very helpful.

In one group, over a 3-month period, a member intermittently appeared with bloodshot eyes and seeming somewhat emotionally labile. One co-leader or the other frequently believed that he was under the influence of Valium, but they rarely agreed about this on any given night. It was thus difficult for them to confront the patient because they found themselves uncertain. Occasionally one or the other would ask him how he was doing with his abstinence or would wonder if the problems he was having had anything to do with his drug use. They always received negative responses. Finally, they brought this to their supervisor and, collectively, the three of them decided that the uncertainty about his status (as well as the intermittent concerns that he might not be leveling with the group) was jeopardizing the patient's effective work in the group. It was decided that the leaders would present this dilemma to him in the group.

They returned to the group the following week and said, "Mr. Stone, for several months now we have wondered off and on whether you might be back on Valium. Last week we both had that concern again. We think it's bad for our relationship with you to be worried about this as much as we are—and also, it must be troublesome to you to have your therapists wondering and doubting. We would like to find a way to resolve this so that the doubt and worry will not stand in the way of work that needs to be done in here. One way that we have thought of to resolve this is that the next time you come to group in a condition that leads one

of us or a group member to wonder about your sobriety, you go down-
stairs to the Inpatient Unit after the group and give a urine sample." The
patient agreed. Though no urines were ever given, the impact of this clear
intervention was that the next week the patient checked himself into an
inpatient program. When he returned to the group he thanked them for
confronting the issue and acknowledged that they had been right all
along.

Regardless of whether urines are an option or not, it is essential
that the group leaders tackle the problem and help define the impasse
that exists. Thus, they may say to the patient, "We're in a very
difficult position here. We know that the group matters a lot to you
and that you want to do the work. But it's terribly important that we
all have faith in what's going on in here and that we all feel good
about the work that we're doing. But I'm wondering how we can do
the work if I'm sitting here wondering and worrying about whether
you're drinking and if you're sitting there wondering about whether
I'm worrying about it. As long as this doubt continues week after
week, it gets in the way of your doing the kind of work that you came
here to do."

The steps involved in dealing with a patient who is actively using
and coming to the group intoxicated involve: (1) empathic enjoinment
with the patient—letting her know that you understand why it's hard
for her to acknowledge her substance use to the group; (2) describing
the impasse—namely, that it is important that you both feel that you
are in a credible relationship, and the way things are shaping up, it
must be very difficult for her to come in week after week having you
doubt her credibility; and (3) problem-solving with the group to get
past the impasse. In the second and third steps the patient (and the
group) is presented with the fact that it is not useful, for the patient or
the group, to be stuck this way, with the therapist wondering and the
patient feeling that the group is on her case each week. The impasse
is put out to the group as a whole, and members are challenged to
think about what can be done about the situation—how they can get
out of the impasse. Thus, the patient is asked, "How can we get out
of the position of wondering each week whether you've been drinking
or not when there's a smell of alcohol in here. What can we do?"
Problem-solving may produce the suggestion of urine screens or a
breathalyzer reading, or some other solution may evolve within the
group.

"Using" and Talking about It with No Intention of Stopping

The patient who continues to drink or use drugs and to let the group know that he does not intend to stop is provocatively defying the group norm. He and the other group members should be asked to discuss their feelings about his continued participation in the group when his behavior so clearly contradicts the basic contract. It is often useful to help the patient see that some part of him wants help and wants to make changes in his life. The struggle that is now being played out in the group (patient behavior in conflict with shared norms and beliefs about what should be happening) is probably a reflection of a similar conflict occurring within the patient himself. It is sometimes helpful for the patient and the group to come to understand this, but more important, the patient (and other group members) must understand that a continued struggle about the basic contract is not productive for either the drinking patient or the rest of the group and cannot go on. The patient may then be asked to decide what he wants to do, and if he feels he cannot make a commitment that is consistent with the group norm, he should be asked to leave.

Continued Use While Verbally Endorsing the Group Norm

The patient who continues to use or who has repeated and frequent slips while at the same time endorsing the abstinence norm usually poses even more difficulty for other group members than does the patient who has no intention of stopping. In fact, the difference between these two patients is probably more a matter of degree than of substance. This patient is not (at least outwardly) struggling with the group at all. She frustrates the group in a more subtle way by continuing to fail. However, since she at least verbally endorses the group norm, it is easier to set up contingency contracts with her. The therapist may say, "It is clear, Mary, that you feel it is appropriate for you to stop using and yet, so far, the ways that you have been dealing with the problem have not been adequate. Since it is important that your behavior, as well as your words, support the group norm, we need to find ways that will be more effective in supporting abstinence." Mary and the group should be asked to set up specific requirements that she will have to follow (e.g., taking Antabuse daily under supervision, going to five NA meetings a week, calling a member of the treatment staff every other day) in order to maintain her group membership.

Regardless of the substance use problem, a number of points need to be kept in mind. The relapsing member who does not endorse the group contract should not be allowed to continue in the group indefinitely. This means that the group leader must assume responsibility for setting limits (or, ideally, getting the group to do so). However, the leader should not lose sight of the fact that he is, in fact, leading a group and that the group needs, and will grow from, a full opportunity to explore each member's own feelings about the patient's behavior, the group's reaction to it, and the patient's departure (if that is how the problem is resolved).

In addition, though there clearly will be times when a patient will have to be helped out of the group, there should be a clear message that the decision is based on his current behavior and that the door remains open for further treatment at a later time. (In some clinics it may even be possible to refer a patient who is unsuitable for group therapy to another counselor with whom he can periodically review his decision about continued use of alcohol or drugs.) It is important to keep in mind that today's relapsing "group failure" may be tomorrow's recovering substance abuser. The way in which he is helped out of treatment at this point may well influence his willingness to get back into treatment in the future.

It should also be remembered that direct confrontation, though sometimes necessary, should be used sparingly and with a clear idea of the intended purpose. The goal of confrontation is not to get the patient "to admit" but rather, to help the patient and the group look squarely at what is going on, with the aim of providing better understanding of the behavior, promoting growth and, when necessary, making changes. Though there will be times (some of these have been outlined above) when direct confrontation is necessary, the therapist who sees his task primarily as learning to invite and encourage discussion will do more to help his group grow than the one who learns only to confront.

Finally, when a member in a group has a "slip"—and particularly if the "slip" becomes a "slide"—it is important for group leaders to listen for material related to other members' feelings about the group and how helpful it is. In addition to feelings of concern, and perhaps anger at the group member who is slipping, members may also feel concerned about themselves and whether they are in a situation that will be adequately containing. Doubts may emerge about the value of the group and the skills of the leader when a member is having a hard time maintaining abstinence.

Need for Outreach

When working with substance abusers, a considerable amount of active intervention by the therapist is needed, particularly in reaching out to "delinquent" patients. The patient who does not show up for a meeting and fails to notify the group in advance, or the patient who leaves a message that he won't be able to make it but whose excuse seems flimsy or ambiguous, needs prompt attention from the therapist. An unannounced absence may be a warning that the patient is in trouble and in some cases may even be a cry for help. For this reason, instead of simply waiting until the next meeting to see what is going on with the patient, it is generally a good idea for the therapist to contact him as soon as possible—right after the group meeting if the patient gave no advance warning, and, if possible, before the meeting if the patient left a message that suggests that with a bit of prompting he might come in.

Although this extra outreach has real advantages in terms of early intervention with patients who may have relapsed, and enables the therapist to cope with potential resistance to treatment, it also has certain disadvantages. In particular, the therapist who consistently reaches out, follows up, and pursues her patients—especially the therapist who communicates disappointment, frustration, or irritation—runs the risk of being perceived by them as taking over the parental role. To avoid this, it is helpful for outreach calls to focus on the patient's behavior (what he may be communicating by his absence, and what he intends to do about his commitment to the group) rather than on the therapist's feelings about the patient's failure to attend.

Communication between Group Leaders and Outsiders

The rules of confidentiality and information exchange are often quite complicated in therapy groups with substance abusers and need to be made explicit as part of the initial treatment contract. The basic rule that what gets discussed within the group is confidential and will not be shared with outsiders is straightforward when it comes to what is expected of the patients. However, in terms of the therapist's contract with her group, there are a number of possible variations that need to be carefully considered.

For example, when a person is referred for treatment by his

employer, with the understanding that continued employment is contingent upon participation in the group (or upon abstinence, or both), the treatment agency may agree to provide information to the employer. If this is the case, the patient must be told in advance that an exchange of information will occur (and a signed release obtained allowing the therapist to talk with the employer). It is important to remember, however, that even when information exchange is part of the treatment plan, a release of information does not give the therapist carte blanche permission to share more than the specifics agreed to. (For example, it would generally not be appropriate to share with an employer personal information about a patient's relationship with his wife.)

Similarly, in some settings there may be an understanding with the family that their continued participation in treatment will be in some way contingent upon their being apprised of the patient's progress. Again, if this is the case, the patient should know exactly what kinds of things the family will be told. (Is it just whether he comes to the group or not, or is there more that will be shared?) Equally important, there should be some indication of what will not be shared.

Finally, in most treatment programs there will be times when one member of the treatment team gets information from a patient that he feels another team member needs to know about. Here, again, patients should be told explicitly what the policy will be. For example, they may be told, "Occasionally, when we feel that it is important to your treatment, information that you bring up in group may be shared with other members of the treatment team. If and when this is the case, we will let you know about it." Alternatively, it may simply be stated that "In our agency we feel that it is important that the entire treatment team know what is going on for you. Thus, whatever you share in the group will be shared, as we feel appropriate, with other staff members in this program."

Equally important as communications to outsiders are communications that come *from* sources outside the group. For example, a patient's husband might call in saying that he believes that she has been drinking, or other patients who are not in the group might let the therapist know that a group member has been "getting high." There are two basic rules of thumb governing the handling of this information. The first is that the therapist make it a policy, explicitly stated, that he will keep no secrets and that any information that he receives will be handled in a manner that he feels is clinically appropriate. He should thus make no promises to patients, spouses, or other family members that what they tell will not be shared. In fact, he should make it clear that the information he receives will be used, as clinically indicated. (And clearly, the concerned other who reports such information does intend that it will have some use.) The therapist receiving the information should not take an oath of confidentiality; to do so ties his hands and puts him in the position of being in collusion with the informant.

The second rule of thumb is that information from outside sources should not necessarily be assumed to be more valid, truthful, or reliable than information supplied by the patient. (Significant others and well-meaning friends can be wrong.) Thus, when the therapist presents information to a patient that he has received from outsiders, his tone should not be "I know you've been getting high because . . ." but, rather, "Your husband called in and was concerned that you might be using again. Can you give us more information about what this is about?" Any discrepancies between the patient's information and analysis of what has gone on and the information that the group leader has received from outside should be pointed out, and the patient should be asked how she understands the discrepancy, or what she makes of it. This is a time when other group members may also get involved, and their attempts to understand what has gone on can be very helpful in cutting through denial.

Finally, it may be helpful to consider the various levels of intervention that may be used in confronting the patient with information from outside the group. It is my belief that the most growth-promoting work that a patient does in therapy occurs when she brings in important and relevant information herself. She should thus be encouraged at first to talk on her own about what is going on, direct confrontation being used only as a last resort. Thus, it is often helpful to begin an intervention, when one feels that a patient's possible alcohol or drug use needs to be addressed, with a general comment such as, "I understand that things have been rough for you the past few days." This is a mild invitation to the patient to speak (and also an indication that the therapist already knows something about what is going on). For many patients this is enough to get them started. Others will tell all about their troubles but will still not acknowledge any drinking or drugging. At this point, the therapist should use directly the information he has from the outside source in the manner described earlier in this chapter (in the section headed "Using but Refusing to Acknowledge It").

Group Focus on Drinking and Drugging

Talking about Substance Use as a Defense against Group Work

It is common in the early stages of group therapy with substance abusers for discussions of alcohol and drug use to predominate. Reminiscences about the "good old days" when "using" was still fun, "war stories" about how bad things finally got, and concerns about current wishes to use (or actual use) pervade the group discussion. Group members establish a sense of cohesiveness by focusing on the one thing—substance abuse—known to be held in common. In addition, though group members have picked a relatively safe way of beginning their involvement in the group, the discussion is, indeed, relevant to one of the stated goals of the group—abstinence.

At times, however, a group may persist in talking about substance use (to the exclusion of all else) long beyond the first few weeks of the group, or may relapse periodically to this limited form of group interaction. When this happens, group leaders often experience a sense of bewilderment—the group feels stuck and is usually dull, yet it appears to be doing what it is supposed to be doing. (After all, what could be more legitimate than discussions about drinking, drugs, AA, NA, etc. in a treatment group for substance abusers?) Another common example of defensive talk about "using" is the following: In the middle of an intense, affectively loaded discussion, a patient interrupts to ask, "What does all this have to do with alcohol or drugs?" His question is heralded by a chorus of support by other group members. The group leader should immediately recognize that this protest is a defense against the painful feelings that are being stirred up in the group and that it expresses a wish to get back onto safer territory. It is, of course, the apparent legitimacy of the drinking/drugging-related talk that makes it such a beguiling group defense against exploring deeper issues and achieving greater intimacy.

Although it is often difficult for the beginning group leader to differentiate defensive talk about drinking and drugging from appropriate discussions of these issues, the two can (and must) be differentiated. Defensive drinking/drugging-related talk is present when any of the following occur: (1) the group seems to talk about little else; (2) the group uses alcohol- and drug-related talk as a distraction, as in the above example; (3) a group member presents an account of a drinking or drugging episode (or a wish to use) that focuses on the details of his thoughts and behavior without attending to the psychological events and feelings associated with the substance use (or the wish to use); (4) the group, in turn, gives advice, or gets distracted with their own war memories.

In contrast, appropriate discussion of drinking and drugging (1) is but one of many topics discussed; (2) is characterized by expression and exploration of feelings; and (3) encourages an exploration of the circumstances (psychological as well as external) that led the troubled group member to feel that he couldn't cope without alcohol or drugs and, if he actually used, what went wrong with the relapse prevention plan and how it was that he had not looked out for himself better.

Finally, while talking about drinking and drugging may be a way for some patients to avoid involvement and intensity, for the patient who feels particularly unworthy it may serve the opposite end. For him, talking about drugs or alcohol may seem like the only "legitimate" way to get a share of the group's time. It is thus essential that the group leader be aware of the many functions of alcohol- and drug-related talk, in terms of both individual and group dynamics.

Drinking and Drugging "In the Service of the Group"

Just as talking about drinking or drugging may serve a defensive function for both the individual patient and the group as a whole, actual alcohol or drug use by one or more members may also serve a function for the group. This is not to imply that the group is a causative agent in the member's relapse, but rather, that her drinking or drugging has an effect on the group that may meet the needs of other group members. Even in a group in which there is a sturdy verbal endorsement of abstinence, a drinking or drugging member may serve several unconscious needs for other group members. First, if the member is still functioning, she reinforces the fantasies held by most recovering substance abusers that some people ("me") can one day "use" again. Her alcohol or drug use may also symbolize the struggle against authority that most groups play out in relation to their leaders in the early stages of group life, or may be used to act out group members' neediness and anger when a group therapist goes on vacation or is otherwise perceived to be rejecting them. Finally, the member who is "using" gives the group a seemingly legitimate reason for continuing to talk about alcohol and drugs—the common safe topic that binds the members together and protects them from the more frightening work of really getting to know one another and themselves.

All of the above factors may prevent the group from tackling the relapsing member's situation in the most productive way and may, at times, subtly reinforce the member's continued use of alcohol or drugs. If the group leaders sense that any of these perpetuation-of-drinking-and-drugging mechanisms may be operating, it may be helpful to share their concerns about it with the group. For example, following the second session in which a patient presents her "drunkalogue" and fellow group members allow (or encourage) it to continue, the leader might say, "I am puzzled at the amount of time the group has spent gathering and listening to details about Martha's drinking. I wonder if her drinking, or at least our talking about it at such length, may serve some function for the group?"

Recovery-Related Defenses in the Individual Group Member

The Patient Who Worries She "May Have to Use"

Occasionally early in group treatment a patient expresses the concern that even though she is committed to abstinence, she has a "personal holdout-contingency plan." For example, a substance abuser who self-medicates when her migraine headaches become serious might state that she feels that if her headaches become severe enough she will probably have to use her Fiorinal. While we might think of this patient as more resistant to treatment than some of our other substance abusers, it is probably safe to say that all of our patients, or at least most, self-medicate to reduce one kind of pain or another (often psychological). And, though most are not explicit about their holdout plans, it is likely that many, if not most, patients reserve the right to use their substance of choice again should things become really intolerable. Thus, the patient (e.g., the migraine sufferer) who expresses this view in the group, rather than being ostracized and left to feel outside of the process, might be enjoined by comments from the group leader indicating that others in the group have also probably maintained the right to have a "personal holdout-contingency plan", and that the thought (wish or fear) that one may fall back on drugs at times of stress or severe pain is probably not unique to her.

The Program Proselytizer

Occasionally, a member enters a group who has had tremendous success with one of the 12-step self-help programs and is disquieted about the presence of others in the group who are not solidly hooked into the program. This member may spend a considerable amount of his time and energy proselytizing about "the necessity of being a regular AA attender and the impossibility of recovering without it," and registering concerns about his own participation in a group where other members are not sufficiently attached to the program. For such individuals, the precariousness of their own recovery and their concerns about maintaining abstinence create tremendous anxiety about the possibility of anyone else deviating from the program that they themselves have embraced. If anyone deviates or fails to be actively involved in the program, it raises the possibility that such deviation is possible. Since, for the avid AA member, his own sense of security about abstinence may be very tightly tied to regular AA attendance, this presents a very threatening specter. With such a patient, it may be useful to underscore that he has learned a lot in AA that has been terribly helpful in maintaining his own abstinence, and *clearly* for him this has been a critical support. While it may be important for the group leader to make it clear that he thinks that AA is a very useful support, the message should also be given that there are other supports that may be useful to others.

The group leader should also consider the possibility that the patient who struggles too ardently on this issue may be setting up a struggle with the group to avoid intimacy. As the group becomes polarized, group process becomes stalemated and group development is halted. In one group that I supervise a particularly graphic example of this occurred.

> All group members had been totally abstinent for many months. Two people graduated who were very staunch AA members, leaving behind one other staunch supporter, two members who attended AA two or three times a week but were not particularly avid program supporters, and two others who did not think AA was very useful. The one ardent member who remained called me in a rage, insisting that I find him a new group where AA would be supported, since, as far as he was concerned, "failing to attend AA regularly was tantamount to having a slip." While initially he created a polarized situation in the group—members trying to convince him that his position was absurd (while he fought

valiantly for the other side)—group members ultimately pointed out to him, "You're afraid of being in here and getting close to us." With the help of the leaders, it became clear that this individual was frightened of remaining in a group situation in which a higher level of intimacy might be achieved. After several weeks of processing the struggle that had ensued (and the group's as well as this individual's willingness to keep the defensive stalemate going), the group was able to effectively move on, with the continued participation of this member (who decided to remain).

The Patient Who Takes the Program Too Literally

For some group members, initial resistance to full engagement in the therapeutic work may take the form of a very literal acceptance of AA's dictum about living in the present and not rehashing the past or "projecting" into the future. It is thus important that the leaders underscore in the pregroup interview, and whenever indicated throughout the life of the group, that the group provides an opportunity to understand how patterns from the past get repeated in the present, as well as an opportunity to examine (and possibly modify) current behavior. In early sessions, "slogan resistance" may first be apparent when leaders ask the group whether members had some thoughts about the previous session, and a member responds, "I just think about what is happening for today. I don't think about the past, and I don't project into the future." This patient is, in a sense, a good student who has learned her lessons well—even if she has taken them a bit literally. To such a patient I might respond, "It's clear that you've learned a lot in AA that's been very helpful to you; and you've learned a lot about the AA ground rules and how that group works. Some of the ground rules in here are a little bit different, though I think you will find that they operate in a complementary fashion."

The Patient Who Obfuscates Through Program Lingo

Often therapists are also confused about how to handle other kinds of "program lingo" (i.e., idioms and slogans from AA, NA, Al-Anon, etc.). Thus, a member in a family program group may say, "Well, clearly I just have 'to let go.'" The group leader, rather than assuming that she understands what the patient is talking about, needs to explore such idioms. Sometimes, the therapist feels as if she should know what the patient means—as if it is a requirement of the therapist working in the substance-abuse field to know and to understand all the idioms and to accept them as complete communications when they come up. Instead, I find it useful to "play dumb" when idioms are used—to act as if I have not yet fully understood what the patient is talking about. Thus, I might say, "How do you mean?" or "Can you say a little bit more about that?" If the patient responds with a tart, "Don't you know what 'letting go' means?" I might respond, "I'm familiar with that expression, but I'm interested in knowing more about what it means in your particular situation." Or I might respond, "Letting go means something a bit different to each person." Basically, the therapist needs to take the same position in terms of making sure that she understands what her patient is talking about when program lingo and idioms are used as she would if a patient were a member of a rare religious sect whose terms were not altogether clear to her. For therapy to be effective, the therapist must be able to tune in to the inner life and experience of the particular patient that she is working with—and to the extent that slogans or labels obscure this, it is important that the therapist not be intimidated by a sense that she "should know what the patient is talking about."

The Patient Who Creates a Sense of "Sameness" through Program Labels

Program labels can also be used to create an illusion of "sameness" to defend against exploring issues in greater depth and against tolerating differences and conflict. Thus, at times of stress in the group, members may attempt to abort further exploration with comments such as, "That's typical alcoholic behavior" or, "This is a typical ACOA issue." Such assumptions about "shared understanding" and "sameness" may create a "you know how it is" mentality in the group, leading to tunnel vision and a reluctance to explore "the obvious." Because the assumption of sameness may prevent the group from moving from one stage of group life to the next, it is important that leaders challenge this assumption when it emerges. A program label should not be accepted as an adequate summary or explanation of what's going on, but rather, should be understood as the patient's attempt to temporarily close the door on painful issues. Thus, when group members summarize what is going on as, "That's typical alcoholic thinking," or "That was a typical ACOA reaction," the leader should ask, "How so?" He should also inquire further about what specifically was going on for the patient involved and what additional kinds of feelings or reactions others in the group might have (thus furthering differentiation rather than supporting the defense of "sameness").

While applying a label to behavior can be helpful in providing a mechanism for conceptualization, premature or inexact labeling may be seen as the kind of defensive soothing that occurs when rationalization is used. Thus, labeling such as, "That's my ACOA behavior," provides a simple surface "explanation" without, in fact, really addressing what is going on. As Bader (1988) points out with regard to the ACOA label,

> . . . labels and catchphrases substitute for real understanding and analysis. A patient will say, "That's my ACA stuff," and invite the therapist to collude under the reassuring pretense that this phrase explains something important, when in actuality it reflects the patient's desire not to analyze what s/he is really feeling. (And). . . short-term relief is purchased at the cost of long-term cure and insight. (p. 98)

Because it is important that labeling not be confused with explaining, when a patient says, "That's my old alcoholic behavior," the therapist should ask for more information by inquiring, "How do you mean?" and then following up with, "What do you make of it?" or, "How do you understand your doing this particular thing?" Too often the process seems to stop once the label has been applied. It is important that group leaders go beyond the naming to find out more about the real phenomenon.

Vulnerability around Holidays

Holidays pose special stresses for all of us—Christmas, our birthdays, and other special holidays are designated as the times when we all want more but often feel that we get less. (Everybody else seems to want more too!) For group members, the holidays also bring up old longings and yearnings for the wonderful times that, often, never were. Childhood wishes for the "perfect birthday" reside in each of us (especially when this wish was never gratified). For many patients, even as adults, it still feels that at least on one day a year—Christmas or one's birthday—everything should work out right. It is important that group leaders tune in to family issues, old yearnings, etc., particularly around holiday time, and assume that in the sessions before major holidays this material is part of what is being talked about even if it is not overtly being stated.

It is also important to recognize that, particularly for substance abusers and their family members, the holiday season poses additional threats because of the massive availability of alcohol. Concerns often come up about how to handle gatherings in one's own home, which has been alcohol-free, when guests are coming who may wish to drink. In addition, the many "invitations to drink" inherent in the easy accessibility of alcohol wherever one turns during the holiday season pose special stress for substance abusers and their family members.

GROUPS FOR COUPLES IN WHICH ONE OR BOTH PARTNERS ARE RECOVERING SUBSTANCE ABUSERS

Treatment of alcoholics and their spouses, both individually and in groups, has received increasing attention in recent years, accompanied by a growing body of research and clinical literature (Cadogan, 1973; Corder, Corder, & Laidlaw, 1972; McCrady, Moreau, Paolino, & Longabaugh, 1982; McCrady et al., 1986; McCrady, Paolino, Longabaugh, & Rossi, 1979; O'Farrell, Cutter, & Floyd, 1985; Paolino & McCrady, 1976; Steinglass, 1979a, 1979b; Steinglass, Davis, & Berenson, 1977; and Vannicelli, 1987). Much of the literature is based on the rationale that the spouse of the alcoholic is seriously affected by the drinking problem, may also be intimately involved in its maintenance, and that couples treatment is the way to maximally impact the dysfunctional marital interactions, as well as the drinking problem itself.

Although there are many similarities between group therapy with couples in which one or both partners are recovering substance abusers and group therapy with other kinds of dysfunctional couples, in the material that follows I highlight some of the themes and issues that seem to particularly differentiate couples groups with substance abusers from couples groups with other populations.*

Communication Issues

In addition to the general advantages of psychodynamically oriented interactional therapy groups outlined in Chapter 2, the couples group

---

*Much of this material is elaborated in an earlier paper (Vannicelli, 1987).

for substance abusers also helps couples learn to communicate with their spouses more effectively.

Communication Problems as a Focus for the Working Alliance

The communication issue is a good place to begin contracting for a working alliance, since communication problems are so frequently present when substance abuse is part of the picture. Communication problems often predate the substance abuse (and perhaps contributed in some ways to it) and are, nearly invariably, introduced or accelerated once substance abuse comes into the picture. It is not just the substance abuser who communicates poorly—those who attempt to interact with someone who is communicating poorly generally find themselves also communicating in maladaptive ways. These dysfunctional patterns from the past continue to be replayed, even when substance abuse is no longer actively part of the system, and need to be unlearned during the process of recovery. Thus, a major focus of the group is to examine the ways that members communicate—what works and what doesn't, both in the group and at home alone with their spouses.

Shaping Between-Session Communications

Since communication problems so often lie at the heart of difficulties that couples experience during the course of recovery and will be a major focus of the couples group, it is useful to begin emphasizing the importance of communication *outside* of the session, as well as *during*, right from the early phases of the therapy. Thus, it may be helpful to say to the couple at the beginning of the second pregroup interview, "What came up during the week as you two talked about our session?" Often patients will respond with something like, "Oh, were we supposed to talk about what happened here? No, we really didn't." I might then inquire gently, "How come?" My question suggests that this is going to be an expected part of the process, and if it does not happen we would want to understand why not. Often the couple's response to this questions is, "We don't talk—about anything—that's part of the problem." I might then ask, "Well, do you think it might be useful to our work if you did talk to one another during the week about some of the things that come up in the group?" The questions that I ask are intended to help shape the couples' expectations regarding the behaviors that will be most conducive to our effective work together.

Disequilibrium Associated with Recovery

The overriding theme in a couples group where one or both partners have had a problem with substance abuse is that abstinence upsets the family and the couple's equilibrium. In much the same way that the alcohol problem might have originally upset the equilibrium, "drying out" also creates changes in the status of the partners relative to one another and a sense that the ground rules have suddenly shifted. A number of studies suggest that, at least in the short run, the resumption of abstinence is often painful for the alcoholic, as well as for members of his immediate family (Vaillant, 1983; Wiseman, 1981; Roberts, Floyd, O'Farrell, & Cutter, 1985). For some couples this may create pressure to reestablish things the way they were—to return to the status quo (drinking and all).

Strangers Starting from Scratch: For many couples there is a sense that they are now two people who do not know each other at all, who are starting over from scratch. Husband and wife may feel like strangers to one another. For some, the distance has not been totally unwanted, and the greater closeness, or potential for it inherent in the new relationship, may be quite uncomfortable or even intolerable. In such cases the couple must often "start over" in terms of getting to know one another. Small steps such as holding hands or taking long walks together may feel like very important first steps to the couple. Often couples (and therapists) feel that the couple "should" have more sexual contact. It must be recognized, however, that the couple is in the process of developing new forms of closeness (e.g., verbal communication, trust) and may temporarily lose other modes (e.g., sexual intimacy) that in the past have been available. If this is the case, the spouses need to be encouraged to feel OK, at least for the time being, with the more limited intimacy that they have newly developed.

Role Change: Many role changes are also associated with recovery. In many families the non-substance-abusing partner will have been the total mainstay for the family, assuming the role of both parents. When the family roles begin to readjust, the overfunctioning spouse may need to give up the role of sole caretaker and "grown-up" in the household. While there may be some gains associated with this, the non-chemical-dependent partner may also experience a sense of loss and may feel abandoned and unappreciated.

The loss associated with the change in roles is sometimes exacerbated further when the chemically dependent member starts seeking support outside of the house, for example, through the use of frequent NA/AA meetings. The spouse of the substance abuser may feel rejected and suddenly in competition with others for the partner's time. To handle this, special negotiation may be required. For example, the two partners may decide to go to AA and Al-Anon on the same night, leaving some other night free specifically for them to do something else together. Contracts about shared time versus unshared time may also need to be made explicit.

The Substance Abuser is the Sick Partner: Another frequent theme among recovering couples is that the non-chemical-dependent person is the "healthy" member, and the chemically dependent one, the "sick" member. Although the non-chemical-dependent partner may also feel and act crazy at times, the flamboyance of the substance abuser's craziness may make it easy for both spouses to blame the substance abuser for the pain they are experiencing. Family, friends, and society at large often contribute to the perpetuation of this myth, looking for some simple mechanism for understanding the couple's distress or for assigning blame. Sadly, however, with abstinence frequently comes the realization that things are as bad between the spouses as ever—only there is no longer a simple explanation. Lost is the explanatory thread (alcohol or drugs) that used to make sense of the longstanding pain. This is often accompanied by another loss—loss of the sustaining fantasy that all would be perfect if only the substance abuser stopped using.

Sometimes an empathic link can be made between the substance abuser and the nonabusing spouse by drawing analogies between the compulsive, out-of-control nature of the substance-abuse problem and some similar problem in the non-substance-abusing partner. For example:

In one couple such a link was made by helping the nonalcoholic spouse to understand his wife's drinking by comparing it to his own impulse-

control problems involving a "short fuse." While the wife complained bitterly about the husband's impulse problems and rageful outbursts, he in turn complained about her drinking episodes and inability to care for herself. The group was able to help them see that in many ways their problems were not so very different. Both at times felt out of control, both had problems that needed treatment, and both behaved in ways for which they felt extremely guilty and that were destructive to a solid relationship.

It is important in running a couples group that both members of the couple understand that they are joining in their own right and that each member of the group is there to work on issues for himself. Spouses are not to join the group as "tag-alongs" because "my spouse thinks it's a good idea." In the same vein, members should be told that they are expected to attend group sessions even if, on a given night, the other member of the couple cannot come. Each person is a valued member of the group, not only as a co-participant with his spouse, but as a separate individual as well.

Differentiating the Couples Group from Al-Anon

As discussed earlier, many members participating in the couples group for substance abusers will simultaneously be members of AA/NA and Al-Anon/Nar-Anon. It is often helpful to discuss the complementarity of the 12-step programs and the couples group in terms of phases or levels of recovery. All substance abusers have a problem with alcohol and/or drugs and, as a first step toward survival, must do something about their substance abuse. AA/NA provides a focus, initially and throughout recovery, on abstinence. Al-Anon similarly focuses on the spouse's survival by helping the spouse "detach" from the substance abusing partner, encouraging her to stop berating the substance abuser or assuming responsibility by covering for his misdeeds. Both AA and Al-Anon also emphasize survival "one day at a time" (as opposed to a long-term future focus). In contrast, the couples therapy group helps recovering substance abusers and their spouses to (1) learn new ways of communicating with one another so that they can cope with their problems together, (2) have a sense of a shared future, and (3) deal with problems that either arose from or were exacerbated by their former patterns of interaction (during the drinking/drugging phase of the marriage). Finally, whereas AA/NA and Al-Anon both encourage members to confide in their sponsors, the couples group emphasizes the importance of learning to confide in one's spouse.

Appropriate Expression of Anger

Understandably, marriages in which there has been substance abuse often accumulate stored-up anger. While spouses may learn in Al-Anon and Nar-Anon that it is not helpful to berate or yell at the chemically dependent spouse for either present or past transgressions, and the meetings themselves may provide alternative mechanisms for letting off steam, leaders must be able to help group members integrate and use their angry feelings productively. The non-substance-abusing partner must learn that there are *effective*, nondestructive ways of communicating anger; this is, of course, important for the substance-abusing partner as well. Moreover, while a litany of complaints from the past is not appropriate, beginning marriage anew on solid footing often requires both members to have some understanding of what has gone on for the other (angry feelings included) during the period of substance abuse.

I would like to underscore and differentiate the kinds of crisis intervention and survival techniques that are important at earlier stages of recovery, namely, "one day at a time," and "detachment," versus the work that can be done once sobriety has been achieved and the couple is striving to have a working marriage. While a building is burning down, one does not stop to inquire how it happened or how participants feel about it. Rescue squads do what they can to blanket the fire and help people escape and protect themselves. Only once the blaze is over and the situation is clearly under control can the event be meaningfully processed and understood.

Use of a Male/Female Co-Therapy Team

In doing a couples group for substance abusers and their spouses, it is especially helpful if a co-leader team can be used. Because of the richness of the couples group and the intricate dynamics that are taking place on many levels—the entire group, each individual, and within the couples themselves—it is especially helpful if there can be two observers to help keep track of what is going on. The co-leaders will benefit from the support they provide one another and the ability to help one another sort things out as they process the group.

Although two leaders of the same sex can be effective, a mixed-sex co-therapy team offers special advantages for the couples group. A male-female co-therapy team can be especially helpful in role modeling the healthy functioning of a couple working together. Frequently, especially in the beginning phases of a couples group, the communications skills of the member couples are so deficient that they cannot serve this function for one another. Thus, the leaders' ability to model adaptive communication, including adaptive ways of disagreeing, may be particularly helpful—role-modeling ways in which a couple clarify and check in with one another. It is often helpful if the co-leaders make a somewhat self-conscious effort to pair in constructive ways in the group. This can be especially helpful in demonstrating ways in which couples can present an allied front and a picture of a working "team" when dealing with other family members. For example, one therapist can make reference to an earlier comment made by the co-therapist as he later elaborates on it. Or one co-therapist can reiterate what the other leader has just said (especially if the message has been a bit confusing) by asking, "Were you saying. . .?" and rephrasing the communication.

Alternatively, the co-leaders may discuss a possible decision openly with one another in front of the group. One leader may say, for example, "I was thinking that one thing we might do is to suggest to Mrs. X that she take a leave of absence from the group until she can resume sobriety and get back on Antabuse. What do you think?" The co-therapist might then respond, "Yes, I think that is a good idea, but it also occurred to me that we might give Mrs. X another week to come back to hear the group's input before we implement that decision." The two co-leaders might then talk about the pros and cons with one another in front of the group, while also asking for the group's input.

Modeling effective disagreement can also be very useful. The co-leaders might actively disagree with one another, either about an interpretation or about the best next strategy. For example, one leader might say to the other, "You were suggesting that Mrs. X might take a leave of absence. I have a different idea that we might consider." Or, "Yes, I can see your thinking there, but I had a very different thought." It is most helpful if these kinds of exchanges communicate that each leader has heard the message of the other, has taken it quite seriously, but may see it from a different vantage point. By showing respect for one another and genuinely processing each other's messages, co-leaders are in a particularly good position to model for the group the ways in which people may disagree without being destructive.

Couples Group Treatment in Combination with Separate Support for Each Member of the Couple

Generally it is helpful if each member of the couple, in addition to being in the couples group, has a separate arena in which to work on his or her individual issues. AA and Al-Anon may be helpful for this, as well as participation in either individual therapy or a group. Although the decision about what kind of additional support and how much is needed will be made on an individual case-by-case basis, if abstinence is precarious, it is especially important that the substance abuser have additional therapy (preferably a substance-abuse group) where he can work on this. If the marriage itself is shaky—and also when the substance abuser's abstinence is precarious—a group for collaterals (discussed in the section that follows) may be particularly helpful for the spouse.

GROUPS FOR COLLATERALS OF SUBSTANCE ABUSERS

This section considers special issues that arise in groups for collaterals of substance abusers—groups for family members and other close associates (which I will also, at times, refer to as family groups). In many settings, these groups are also referred to as relatives groups, significant-other groups, or co-dependency groups. (The latter term I tend not to use because of its increasing ambiguity.) I differentiate these groups from ACOA groups (which are, of course, also for family members) based on proximity to the substance-abuse conflict (the crisis hierarchy referred to in Chapter 3). Groups for collaterals are intended for those who are currently living with substance abusers (or those in recent recovery)—the partners and parents, and sometimes the grown children, if they are still actively involved in the day-to-day life of the active or recently recovering substance abuser. This is differentiated from the ACOA group (discussed later in this chapter), where there is less immediacy to the present substance-abuse issues of the parents.

Although there is some research data to suggest that the treatment of family members may have a positive impact on the substance abusers' drinking or drug use (Wright & Scott, 1978), the focus of our groups for collaterals is not on the substance abuser. Rather, these groups are designed to help foster the emotional growth of family members who often experience considerable pain and despair as they attempt to cope (often ineffectually) within a dysfunctional family system. These groups help family members to better understand the parts they play in perpetuating their untenable life situations and to assume responsibility for improving the quality of their own lives.

"I Am Not the Problem"

Often, the presenting issues for collaterals involves them in a self-presentation that may seem antithetical to doing any therapy work at all. Namely, they see the chemically dependent spouse or grown child as "the problem"—seeing themselves as "the victim." They may even be reluctant, initially, to call themselves "patients" or to engage in any activity that is referred to as "therapy." Yet, they are clearly in pain, and the therapist's job is to align with them around this so that relief may ultimately be possible.

Entrenchment in the Quagmire of Despair

These patients are also frequently stuck—peculiarly entrenched—having developed coping mechanisms for survival which have, indeed, helped them to survive, but which may also be difficult to give up. For many family members, patiently standing by has led to standing still—anchored, like the rock of Gibraltar, for so long that the possibility of movement seems remote.

The weight of the hopelessness and despair that these family members live with can, at times, drag the group leaders along with them into the quagmire—leaders and members alike feeling unable to move. The skilled leader needs to understand the depth of this entrenchment and to be sensitive to her own countertransference reactions when she feels pulled in. In addition to helping the group understand (through the kind of projective identification interpretations discussed in Chapter 10) that she is now feeling the same way that members often feel, the leader must also be skilled at promoting an exploratory attitude that at least keeps open the possibility of future movement. These group members may take longer to actually begin their journey, but progress can be made toward this end as long as the leader encourages interest in getting on board and continues to examine resistance to making changes.

At times such a group may unwittingly serve the purpose of aiding and abetting resistance; it allows itself to become just a comfortable place where people commiserate with one another. Group members may become entrenched with a group of others who understand and are sympathetic (as is sometimes the case with Al-Anon and ACOA meetings, where many go not so much to change as to find a modicum of comfort in the untenable situation that they are living in). This is probably, in some ways, a good use of Al-Anon. But in a therapy group we hope for more than this. We can help the group to achieve more by focusing on what each member was hoping to get when he joined the group and what he feels would have to happen in the group in order for this to occur.

It is also helpful at times to point out to group members that although there is a part of them that wants to make certain kinds of changes, there is another, perhaps equally powerful part, that would find it frightening to do so. Thus, it is helpful to talk about the scared part that may want to keep things as they are. The leader can help group members talk about their resistance by asking, for example, "What do you suppose it is that keeps you living in the situation the way that it is?" To this the patient may respond, "Nothing! Who would want to live in such a situation?" To this the leader might respond, "And yet, it continues, so there must be some kind of reinforcer or some things about it that we need to understand more about. One reinforcer that keeps us from changing is that the familiar often feels more manageable than the unknown."

In our clinic, the groups that seem to get the most entrenched—where the group resistances at times seem to overpower the forces for change—are the family groups. Whereas ACOAs come with an agenda to work on their family-of-origin issues and move quickly to a level of engagement with the past in an effort to understand its application in the present, and substance abusers have an immediate goal of making at least those changes necessary to maintain abstinence, family members are often more confused about the group's task and their own personal goals. Are they there to learn how to better tolerate an intolerable situation? (A somewhat entrenched position.) Are they there to make changes? If so, in whom? Some family members join, in fantasy, to make changes in somebody else—to "get him to change." Although this is not a realistic therapy goal, it may be the hidden agenda for some of our patients.

"I Am Overwhelmed": A Signal That the Work Has Begun

Other family members, particularly those who are entering treatment for the first time, may within the first few sessions experience the feeling of being "overwhelmed." They are in a new situation that poses the possibility of making changes and discovering things about themselves that may be frightening. The "overwhelmed" feeling may be a familiar one—the feeling which for many people from dysfunctional families has signalled the "turning-off" adaptation that becomes a part of how they relate to their intimate worlds. Often when the patient begins to experience this, it is accompanied by the feeling that perhaps the group is not for him. However, this first feeling, while sometimes scary, should not be seen as a sign that the patient should quit, but rather, as a positive harbinger that the work has begun. It is often helpful, in fact, to let patients know that the fact that they are experiencing some anxiety is an indicator that they are right on track. The next step is for them to learn that these feelings can be tolerated (even though the patient's initial reaction is "I am overwhelmed—I need to pull out or pull back") and that the feelings will be manageable as they are understood through the work in the group. Thus, patients learn that when they feel overwhelmed, "turning off" is no longer the only available solution.

The Patient Who Talks Only about Her Substance-Abusing Significant Other

The patient who joins a group for family members is often unclear about the task of the group and her role in it. Although attempts to clarify this should be made to group members as early as the pregroup interview, confusion often continues (aided by resistance), and periods of clarity about the group's goals may be temporarily lost during periods of individual or group stress. Confusion about the group's task (and/or resistance) most commonly manifests itself by group members focusing primarily on their lives outside of the group, in particular on the substance-abusing significant other. Often, week after week is spent in lengthy diatribes that produce relatively little new information (about the patient or her significant other) and often lull the group into a stupor.

To help members develop a more viable role in the group, leaders can encourage members to reflect on what they are doing in the group and the utility of their behavior in terms of the goals that they have outlined for themselves. Thus, the leader might ask, "What are you hoping for in sharing this material about your husband?" or, "How are you hoping the group will help with this?" Frequently, the patient's initial response is a somewhat blank, confused reaction: "Gee, I don't know, I'm not sure I was expecting anything." The therapist, aiming to help the patient understand that her participation in the group will ultimately be the most helpful if it is, indeed, purposeful, might ask, "Well, what was your understanding of what we would be doing here?" The patient again may respond with confusion, or may say, "I don't know—aren't we supposed to be talking about our spouses?" The therapist can use the patient's confusion as a springboard to clarifying the group's task, by asking, "Well, if group members mostly talk about their substance-abusing husbands and wives, how much do you think members will learn about themselves?" and, "What other things do you think might be useful for the group to talk about?" He might also ask group members, "What do you remember about this from what we talked about in the pregroup interview?"

The leader's task, thus, is to help patients reflect on how the group can be useful to its members and whether the way the group is currently functioning will serve its members most effectively. It is important to remember that patients are often confused for long periods of time about what therapy, and in particular group therapy, is all about; and the therapist's questions are a way of helping patients to formulate a clearer sense of the group's purpose. (Toward this end, of course, it is also essential that the therapist himself have a clear idea of the task at hand and the goals that he has for the particular kind of group work that he is doing.)

One important goal of a psychodynamically oriented interactional therapy group is to think about its utility in helping patients better understand their own emotional lives and the pushes and pulls that motivate them. Group therapy also helps members to appreciate the complexity of human relationships by providing a clearer view of how members react to others, and how at times they sabotage the kind of connections they most want. Clearly, these tasks will be only minimally addressed if the group stays focused on outside-of-group material. The group task will be more fully accomplished the more outside-of-group material can be tied to the here-and-now process in the group as a way of exploring the characteristic ways that the patient relates to his world.

A Substance Abuser within the Context of a Group for Collaterals

In the course of group work with family members, a substance-abuse problem may be revealed among one of the group members. Once we learn that a group member has a chemical dependency problem, it is important that we see to it that an appropriate treatment recommendation is made.

> In one group the leader, along with the group members, learned that a member was abusing tranquilizers—and had been for some years. The group did not tackle the issue, and the leader, hoping that his gentle prods would help the group to move in a productive direction with the chemically dependent patient, failed to take definitive action himself. Of course, part of the difficulty for the group was that these family members had, for years, lived with people who were chemically dependent—often feeling angry, helpless, and unempowered to do anything about it. Since it is likely that the same feelings were being recapitulated in the group, the leader found it difficult to enlist the support of group members without taking a more active stand himself. After discussing the situation with his supervisor, the leader let the group member know that, in order to achieve the goals the patient had set for herself in the group, she would need to be chemically free. Thus, if she wished to remain in the group to work on the difficulties she was finding living with a chemically addicted husband, she needed, in addition, to join a group where she could work on her own substance-abuse problem.

In such instances, it is essential to move clearly and quickly with the chemically dependent member to be sure that she gets treatment for her own substance-abuse problem. If she wishes to remain in the relatives group along with a substance-abuse treatment group, this might remain an option—depending on how other members of the group feel about it. And the feelings of other members do need to be actively explored, since a family members group may feel "invaded" by having a chemically dependent member among them.

Referring such an individual to individual therapy or sending her to AA is generally not adequate. With regard to individual therapy (unless the focus is specifically on relapse prevention), weeks may go by without talking about substance abuse. In contrast, if the member joins a substance-abuse group, this issue is always potentially part of the agenda (even if it is on a back burner); the patient's presence in a substance- abuse group—her return each week to a setting in which all members are committed to abstinence and to talking about wishes to use, as well as actual slips, keeps the focus on substance abuse.

With regard to AA, there is generally no way of ascertaining if the patient actually attends or not. There may be some exceptions to this—for example, a patient who has already had a long, successful history with AA and has used it reliably as a support, or one who has a sponsor in AA who will help keep her plugged in and help with accountability. But otherwise, simply referring a resistant patient to AA and hoping for the best is often not adequate treatment for the substance-abuse problem. In my view there is nothing like a substance-abuse group to keep the patient focused on these issues.

What the therapist might say to such an individual is, "Clearly this is an issue that you are familiar with—having lived with a chemically dependent person for so many years yourself; it is also clearly an issue that the entire group is familiar with. It is essential that you now make sure that your own substance-abuse problem is being addressed in order for you to do the work in here. It doesn't make sense for us to pretend that you can examine the impact of your husband's addiction on you and your family when you're not focusing on your *own* addiction. It is thus important, if you want to continue the work in here, that you have a solid platform to stand on; that means that you have to get specific help for your own substance abuse."

The patient should be given a week or two to think about it and talk about it in the group and then should be discharged from the group unless the substance-abuse treatment group has been embraced. Particularly in a relatives group, it is important to act firmly and expeditiously with regard to this issue, since the leader is working with a room full of group members all of whom have been in precisely the same dilemma—often for many years (namely, having to contend with someone close to them who needs substance-abuse treatment). Thus, the leader's role-modeling is essential in taking a clear position about the need to address the substance abuse before any other work can be effectively done.

GROUPS FOR ACOAs

Although the "core constellation" of the adult-child "syndrome" remains empirically undocumented, what does seem to be shared, at least by those ACOAs who find their way into treatment, is an awareness that their family lives were dysfunctional in significant ways that now affect their adult functioning. While such a view of oneself and one's family of origin is no doubt shared by members of many other clinical populations who have grown up in dysfunctional families, what may be special for the ACOA is that the current focus on this form of family dysfunction may provide, for the first time, a sense that his problems can be labeled and remediated.

The ACOA movement, and in particular the presence of ACOA groups, provides an opportunity for many adults from dysfunctional families to find a way into treatment. The sense that "something is wrong," that others may share similar problems, and that family-of-origin problems from the past are the cause of current problems in relating to others and in living full lives, are all brought into focus by the growing ACOA movement. For many, the ACOA focus provides a comfortable entree into treatment that might otherwise not be available (see Vannicelli, 1989, 1990, 1991, for fuller elaboration of these issues).

Intense "Family Dynamics" and Transference

Part of the glue for initial and continued bonding in ACOA groups is the shared presenting issue regarding the ACOA identity. This homogeneity around the presenting issue continues to create greater intensity within the group than is often true of more heterogeneous groups because there is less diffusion of focus. In heterogeneous therapy groups, some patients present around issues with parents, others around dysfunctional behavior in the workplace, others present with feelings that have been stirred up over the loss of a loved one, and others with diffuse anxiety or depression. Moreover, members enter at different stages of awareness regarding the importance of past family experiences in understanding their current presenting issues. It sometimes takes months—even years—for patients to link up their present difficulties to issues in their families of origin (and there is often considerable resistance to doing this). The diversity among members provides more ready distraction from the intense family-of- origin and transference issues that are ultimately part of any therapy group. In contrast, in the ACOA group all members come with the knowledge that their work involves rethinking issues regarding their past relationships in their families of origin and how these issues relate to the present. Although members may vary considerably in terms of level of sophistication and clinical awareness, the family is a more ready focus for the overt content of the group, and family transference is more readily enacted.

Thus, the themes described in the following material are likely to take on special meaning in ACOA groups because they recapture the family dynamics of *several* members—with a greater number of group members lending themselves to the group enactments that emerge (and fewer members left to provide observing ego). It is thus especially important that the leader is prepared for these themes, understands what is going on, and is able to provide a healthy observing ego, when necessary.

The powerful family transference that develops in all dynamically oriented therapy groups is particularly potent in these groups for a number of reasons. First, many ACOAs fear, as they first enter treatment, that in talking about family "secrets" they are in some way abandoning or betraying their families of origin (Beletsis & Brown, 1981). This is often further complicated by a longstanding (and forbidden) wish to be able to separate emotionally (or even physically) from their families. There are thus conflicting feelings involving betrayal and abandonment, as well as a healthy wish to separate.

The fear that, by entering therapy and making changes, the ACOA will be abandoning (or abandoned by) the family of origin makes the entry into a new "family" (the group) an even more intensely loaded venture. As Brown (1988) suggests, transference thus develops quickly and often intensely, as members embrace the new family that, at least in fantasy, will replace the one they are leaving behind. Along with this, the group leaders also become powerful transference figures—and often, initially, highly idealized. There is an understandable hope and wish that the leaders will provide the good (perhaps perfect) parenting that was absent in childhood, and that the group will be the close and supportive family long yearned for. This conscious idealization of the family group tends to be even more prominent than in more heterogeneous therapy groups—in part because it is more likely to meet a shared and salient need of many of the members.

However, the power of the positive idealization (the initial cement of the group) also carries with it the seeds of its obverse—negative transference and feelings of intense disappointment. In other words, the powerful, initial family fantasies create rapid bonding and lead to greater initial investment. However, along with this there may also be greater intensity of negative feelings, including tremendous fear of disappointment—and often actual disappointment. As we shall see, this intense initial chemistry relates substantially to most of the themes that follow.

Flight from the Group (The Wish to Leave Prematurely)

The wish to leave an ACOA group is an ever-present theme, and threats to leave or run away are frequently expressed, in terms of wishes either to flee from the session or to terminate from the group. The fantasied solutions of the past ("escape" from the pain and conflict) are thus reenacted in the ACOA group over and over again as conflict is encountered and as tensions rise. Because there was no doubt a time for many ACOAs when the fantasy of running away was all that sustained them, it is not surprising that group members continue to think about it (and even attempt to enact it) as a solution in the new family (the group) as well. The leader's task is to help group members understand that their wish represents a fantasied solution of the past, but that they are now in a situation in which there are constructive alternatives to fleeing.

It should also be noted that the wish to flee, in addition to being a familiar solution to old family conflicts, may also emerge because of new feelings that are being stirred up. Even the "positive" feelings regarding the "perfect" parents and the wonderful, close family can be very frightening for those members who have had little experience regulating closeness and intimacy.

Finding (and Removing) the Identified Family Problem

Although scapegoating may occur in any group, ACOA groups are often especially inclined to pick "an identified patient" (IP), whom the group may first "try to cure," ultimately decide is "too sick," and finally attempt to extrude. As in most instances of scapegoating, the chosen IP complies in some way, as he shares the group fantasy and lends himself to its enactment. In this instance, the collective myth is that the family will finally be restored to happiness when the "problem" is removed. In other words, the group enacts the cherished fantasy of childhood that the idealized family will finally occur if the troubled (alcoholic) member is gone. In fact, the group may move from one member to another, attempting to discover "who is the sickest," in order to target the identified patient so that the group can either cure or extrude him and thereby restore the health of the family.

The Search for a Rescuer

Closely related to the group's search for the "problem" patient is the search for a grand and powerful figure who will "come to the rescue." While initially this wish may be projected onto the group leaders in the form of idealized transference, as the group moves on (and particularly as the group leaders come to be viewed more ambivalently), the members may look for a "rescuer" among themselves. The patient who is assigned this role (and who, often, all too willingly complies) may then become as rigidly stuck in this position as the identified patient may become in his.

It falls to the group leaders in both instances (with the scapegoated "identified patient" and the assigned "hero") to help the group understand its need to have these roles filled, and also to understand the ways in which the designated actors comply. In the case of scapegoating, it is sometimes helpful for the leader to ask if the identified patient might in some way be "serving a function for the group." If the group has difficulty responding, the leader may help further by commenting, "I have a hunch that the group's view of Sam as 'the sick one'—perhaps too sick for this group—might be helpful to the group in recreating some old, familiar patterns. I wonder if it's possible that the group's wish to cure him or get rid of him might feel like a solution that could be understood from the past."

Similar questions to the group about the role of the rescuer might be as follows: "It seems as if the group has a powerful wish to see Susan as the 'rescuer' in here. I wonder if her portrayal of herself as so much healthier than the other group members, and the group's readiness to buy this, might serve some function for the group." After exploration, the leaders may again share their hunches about the possibility that the group is enacting something in the present that might have seemed like a solution in the past. And again, although the entire group's involvement in the enactment will be important, the particular individual's willingness to play a particular role should also be explored.

Rigid Role Assignments

In both of the themes illustrated above (scapegoat and rescuer), it is clear that group members may find themselves solidly entrenched in specific, relatively limited roles, with the collusion and support of the group. Although, to some extent, this dynamic is possible in all psychodynamically oriented therapy groups, it may be exaggerated in ACOA groups because dysfunctional families may be particularly likely to develop stereotyped and rigid roles that keep the family system in balance. A series of research studies (Davis, Berenson, Steinglass, & Davis, 1974; Steinglass, 1979a; Steinglass et al., 1977) have documented that alcoholic families display a more rigid interactional style than is the case with nonalcoholic families, and that family members tend to act in more rigidly coordinated patterns, particularly during alcohol-free periods. Although there is no empirical validation to date for the particular kinds of roles that individuals may play, there is some research that suggests, at least, a certain level of role constriction and stereotypy of response—perhaps due in part to a need to increase predictability in an arena in which this is frequently lacking. The quest for predictability may manifest itself similarly in the ACOA group, where again people may fall into predictable roles with regard to one another and with regard to the group.

Hanging On

Although less common than the theme of flight, another theme that reenacts a part of the old family drama is tenacious "hanging on."

Some patients, even after they have finished the work they initially came for, find that they cannot leave. Termination dates are repeatedly set and put off. The final piece of work for these patients (often a substantial task) involves helping them to understand the difficulties they have in letting go.

For such patients, many of whom lived much of their childhoods in hopeful anticipation that things might one day get better, hanging on has become a dysfunctional solution. They continue to live with the persistent feeling that if they hang on a little longer, the longed-for "pearl" will finally be delivered. They are unable to leave the group because they cling to the old fantasy that with a little more time and a little more effort, a lot more will be forthcoming. Such patients have difficulty separating from the group (and often separating from inappropriate people in their lives outside of the group) because they cannot let go of the hope that, with steadfast persistence, Cinderella's wish (the yearned-for connection, closeness, and caring) will finally come true. Such patients live with the fantasy, which they repeatedly reenact, that the people that they love will one day return the caring measure for measure, and that if they just hang in long enough and do enough, they will finally get what they have held out for. This is replayed over and over as the patient continues to chose love objects who can never fully acknowledge love or love back in return. Such patients continue, often throughout repeated relationships, to "turn somersaults" in order to get what seems not to be forthcoming.

These patients need to understand that these fantasies, while offering great "staying power," often prevent them from getting their needs met from other more appropriate sources. People, including group members and group leaders, have their limits. The fantasy of what one "should have gotten" and is still holding out for may not be in keeping with what is realistically available. To help such patients terminate from the group, it is often necessary to help them understand the real limitations that existed in past relationships, and the group's limitations as well.

The Problem Is Outside of Me

As noted previously, the ACOA focus provides patients, particularly initially, with a focus outside the self. For many patients, externalization is a comfortable and preferable alternative to the self-blame that they have carried for years. For some, it appears that there is now an understandable "cause" for their problems. Thus, particularly in the early phases of group life, there may be considerable focus on blaming the parents (both the parents of childhood and the parents of the present, who continue to perpetuate the crimes of the past). Along with this, group members may spend time focusing on ways to change members of their families of origin and may find it difficult to focus on themselves. When this happens, it may be useful for group leaders to refocus the group with comments such as, "The family members who are not present in this group seem to get considerably more attention than those who are here. My hunch is that the troublesome family members that we are hearing so much about have always gotten more than their fair share of the attention. What would it be like for the family members who are here if more of the focus were to be on you?"

Negative Self-View to Preserve Parental "Goodness"

Early and unmet needs for love and support may lead not only to dysfunctional relationships but also to a dysfunctional negative self-identity. The need to believe that parents are "good" and "loving" is basic to a child's sense of safety and security. When reality challenges this basic assumption, the child from a dysfunctional family may alter beliefs about himself to protect parental goodness and integrity (Brown, 1988; Wood, 1987). Simply stated, if a child perceives himself as "bad," he justifies parental neglect and even abuse by his otherwise "good" parents. As Brown (1988) states, "The child experiences the absence or loss of parental attention as a response to something bad about the child . . . (thus providing) an illusion of security because it leaves the parents intact as available and caring figures and places the responsibility for problems on the child" (p. 132).

Wood (1987), succinctly summarizing the thinking of the British object relations theorists (Fairbairn, 1943/1981; Guntrip, 1969; Winnicott, 1955/1975), adds to our understanding of this important dynamic:

> . . . when children cannot build satisfying relations with their parents—because the parents are abusive, neglectful, or both—the children try to achieve a sense of control over their terrifying predicament by internalizing those aspects of the parents that seem most

frightening and destructive. . . . These psychic maneuvers permit children to maintain an illusory sense of control over a threatening situation, but because the bad objects are installed in the psyche and become part of the self, they have devastating effects on self-esteem. (p. 29)

The ACOA Label

For many ACOAs, another aspect of negative self-identity may include the ACOA label itself. Although identification of oneself as an ACOA has many positive aspects, particularly in terms of feeling that one's problems can be understood and remediated, overattachment to one's "ACOAness" may ultimately impair growth by perpetuating a negative self-view. As one group member put it when he began to form healthier relations with peers, "I no longer wish to have so much of my world view focused on my ACOAness."

As discussed earlier, in the process of identity formation, the child, attempting "to spare his parents" and keep them as "good" as possible, in exchange may take on bad or negative views of himself. These bad parts become an important part of the identity of the ACOA. It is thus important to keep in mind that an overly salient identity as an ACOA may reflect not a healthy adaptation but, rather, a need to cling to a bad view of oneself in order to keep the world in balance.

An ad in the "personals" section of *Boston Magazine* captures the salience of an ACOA identity for one particular individual. It began: "DWF 46 FRIEND OF BILL W's, ACOA, nonsmoker, loves humor. . . ." This ad, I think, reflects the enormous importance of the ACOA identity to this individual and her wish to preserve it in subsequent relationships with significant others. She was putting out a sign, unconsciously inviting those who would pair with her "defective" part (and continue to reinforce it) to join her in a relationship.

An important goal of group therapy is to put the ACOA identity in its proper perspective. That one's parents were alcoholic is a to-be-accepted fact. The ACOA's picture of himself will always involve this fact, and through the course of therapy it will help explain many aspects of the patient's past. Brown (1988) indicates that for many ACOAs ". . . the most significant change begins with the acquisition of the identity ACA"—the first step in "making real the past" (p. 291). Yet ideally, with successful therapy and the emergence of a more positive and more integrated self, the centrality of the ACOA identity will recede.

Resistance to "Taking a Look" at What's Going On

Because children who grow up in dysfunctional families often get messages from their parents that seem to invalidate the child's perception that something is wrong, a coping strategy is sometimes developed of "not seeing" what's happening. Children from alcoholic families who confront their parents about drinking problems may be told that there is "no problem," or they may even be given the impression that they are "bad" for noticing. Thus, for many ACOAs, the experience of feeling uncomfortable about what's going on, but not feeling that they have either permission to really look at it or to voice their concerns, may be a common experience. Sometimes this will become apparent in the group when members have difficulty actually looking at one another or at the therapists; at other times it may become apparent when an individual group member or the group as a whole appears to have difficulty taking a real look at what's going on in the group itself. At such times, it may be helpful for group leaders to suggest to the group that "members seem to feel that in some ways they do not have permission to really 'see' what's happening," and to suggest that this might be something that the group might want to take a better look at. Members, through the process of their group work, thus may have an opportunity, for the first time, to go back and take a look at their past experiences and to see them as they really were. At the same time they have an opportunity in the group to learn to look at how things really are in the present and to learn to trust their perceptions of reality.

Concerns about Predictability of Authority Figures

In the early stages of group life, members often express "curiosity" about the group leader and her past—particularly about whether the leader herself is an ACOA. The question relates, in part, to patients' concerns about whether the therapist will be able to understand and to help. In addition, it often reflects concern about whether the therapist has had the same kind of unpredictable parenting that they have had—and whether, in turn, the therapist will replicate that erratic parenting in the group, as some members find themselves doing in relation to their own children. Even the positive, initially good therapist (the idealized leader) may come to be viewed with suspicion. Group members may feel, "You've been good tonight, active, responsive, done things the way we like—but will you stay this way beyond the first few sessions?" It is as if members are communicating that they do not want to count on something that will disappear. Their own concerns about inconsistent parenting are thus projected onto the leader, with the particular worry that the leader may be as inept as their own parents (and as they may be with their own children). For the ACOA who has experienced inconsistency in parenting, the question may periodically resurface regarding how consistent the leader will be, since even good things often turn bad.

Concerns about consistency and predictability of the leader can be addressed, in part, by the general demeanor of the leader with regard to consistency (as discussed in Chapter 10 with regard to limit setting, clear boundaries, etc.). Many leaders may also be tempted to answer questions about their ACOA status directly. However, whether one answers or not, it is essential to take up the underlying concerns that are being expressed.

Concerns about Early Problem Drinking

Unlike many alcoholics, who are often the last to be aware of the severity of their problems with alcohol, ACOAs may have a heightened sensitivity regarding potential problematic use of alcohol and other drugs. Often, even when friends and family are unconcerned about the quantity and frequency of the ACOA's substance use, the ACOA will be worried and anxious about her use of chemical substances. Thus, for example, some ACOAs may find themselves drinking only an occasional beer—but when their quantity exceeds this even slightly (e.g., occasions on which they might have two drinks), or when they find themselves doing this more than once or twice a week, they feel quite concerned about their potential for alcohol abuse. Although abstinence is not necessarily the only appropriate solution for these ACOAs, when the situation has come up in our groups, members have often been effective in helping such individuals either to abstain or to set limits on their drinking that they feel more comfortable with. It may also be useful for the leaders to ask why, if the drinking seems to cause such discomfort, the person continues to drink.

This chapter has examined some of the special issues and themes that are likely to be particularly salient in groups for substance abusers, groups for collaterals, couples groups where one or both members are recovering substance abusers, and ACOA groups. These special issues are put into a broader context in subsequent chapters as we more fully explore the group's journey and the many roadblocks that may be encountered along the way.

❖ 6 ❖
Defining the Journey

Despite the fact that we refer particular populations of patients to groups that have specific nominal themes, such as recovery groups, family members groups, ACOA groups, these group labels neither limit nor adequately define the work that is to be done. The central task of group therapy—regardless of patient population—is to help the patient better understand her feelings, thoughts, and wishes, how she communicates them, and how this affects her ability to connect with others in a meaningful way. The group provides a safe arena in which important aspects of members' interactions with others are replayed and can be productively examined, understood, and modified. To achieve this, the group, with the help of the leader, must:

1. *Provide support.* This is essential for creating a safe context for the therapeutic work in general, and may take on special importance when the group or a particular member is in crisis and extra containment is needed.
2. *Attend to "here and now" process within the group.* Much of the benefit of group therapy derives from the opportunity to examine what goes on in the group as a way of understanding the ways in which members relate to important people in their lives and the interpersonal situations they get themselves into. The group thus becomes a forum for enacting important conflicts and interpersonal issues.
3. *Examine past antecedents (historical roots).* The group provides a unique arena in which to observe (and understand) the ways in which the past is replayed in the present. An opportunity is thus afforded for integrating past and present.

A key variable shaping the success of the group's journey is the leader's understanding of what is to transpire and how these three group activities will be used to complement one another. This is explored in Chapter 10 as we examine some of the confusion that often exists for the therapist regarding the leader's role and clinical stance.

In the material that follows I address several issues important for understanding the substance and style of dynamically oriented interactional therapy groups—issues that are more global thematically than the population-specific issues in the preceding chapters, or the group, patient, and therapist roadblocks that are dealt with in Chapters 7, 8, 9, and 10.

Underscoring Use of the Group as a Forum for Enacting Important Conflicts and Interpersonal Issues

To help focus group members so that they can understand (and will be thinking about) the ways in which important aspects of their interaction with people outside the group are replayed in the group, specific questions can be helpful. These might include some of the following. "In what ways do you think that you play out in here the kind of things that are hard between you and your wife (mother, boss, etc.)?" If the patient says, "I think there's a little bit of this in my relationship with Susan," the group has an opportunity to explore that particular interaction as it unfolds in the group—shedding light on important issues and conflicts for both of these group members.

If, on the other hand, the patient responds rather blandly to the question, "Does any of the sort of thing you are talking about come up in here?" the therapist may have a chance to be somewhat educative. Thus, for example, if the patient responds by saying, "No, nothing like that does come up in here—should it?" the therapist might respond, "One of the ways that this kind of therapy works is that the group becomes an arena in which the characteristic ways that members relate to people on the outside (outside of group) can be looked at. When the group is working at its very best, we have a chance to use the group as a sort of minimicrocosm in which we can see and come to understand how people's issues unfold." Of course, it is important that the therapist herself understand that this is how therapy works. Therapy, whether individual or group, is not effective simply because patients "report." Rather, the work of the therapy gets done through transference reactions to both the therapist and other group members, allowing important aspects of the patient's conflicts to get played out in the group.

A bland response that denies any similarity between behavior in the group and behavior outside may be explored further by additional questions from the therapist, such as, "The kind of thing that you have been describing really does seem to happen quite a bit with people who are important to you. What is it, do you suppose, that's different in here that makes this kind of thing not come up?" The response to these questions may shed light on the ways in which the patient limits his interactions in the group and controls his affective range to preclude the group's fully coming to know parts of him.

In any case, even if no immediate pay dirt comes from questions in this arena, such questions are a reminder to the individual patient, and to the group as a whole, that when group therapy is working effectively, the group does become a screen on which important issues, conflicts, and styles of interaction get replayed and in which they can be examined and understood by the group.

Clarifying the Focus: Dealing with Group Confusion about the Journey

In Chapter 8 we discuss strategies that members may use to pull the group away from meaningful exploration of interactions in the here and now and to dilute progress toward group bonding and cohesion. Sometimes similar behavior may stem, at least in part, from confusion about the group contract—the defensive forces in the group being aided and abetted by confusion about what is actually supposed to take place. Thus, when a group member proclaims that she is dissatisfied because the group is not doing enough of one thing or another, it is important to understand the patient's conception (or misconception) about what should be happening.

Complaint in a Substance-Abuse Group That There Is Too Little "Recovery Talk"

In an early-stage group, where some members are still having trouble with sobriety, or at a later stage when a member has slipped, much of the group focus will appropriately involve recontracting with the slipping patient and understanding her failure to use adequate supports. At such times, a "recovery focus" is indeed appropriate. But what about a group in which all members have been abstinent for some period of time? Confusion about the need for a recovery focus reflects lack of clarity about the group contract; and such confusion can only be sorted out if the leader, himself, has a clear idea about what it is he hopes will happen in the group.

It is important that the therapist keep in mind that even in early recovery groups, the goal is to help people understand more about themselves. To the extent that we can transmit this understanding to our patients, we provide a fuller and more interesting focus for group life than were the group to limit itself to discussions of "recovery." The following vignette illustrates both patient and therapist confusion about this important issue.

A group member who had been stably abstinent for over a year began complaining 10 months after joining the group that there was too little talk about "recovery issues." The group leader, whom I was supervising, indicated that he thought his patient might be right—since, indeed, the group had not talked for a long time about "recovery." As he spoke about his concerns, it became clear that he, himself, was uncertain as to what the group should be doing or whether what members were currently doing (working on interpersonal relationships within the group) was appropriate. Yet surely it was, since recovery in the fullest sense must attend to the quality of people's interactions with others.

When we think about this in a more folksy way, it is useful to consider the fact that people's substance abuse is nearly always, in one way or another, intricately related to "what's the matter with them"— "the stuff that doesn't work." Either their "stuff" is causally linked to begin with (and is part of what got them into trouble with chemical substances) or, even if not originally causally connected, their current problems become stressors that strain against maintaining abstinence. Behavioral conceptualizations of substance-abuse recovery, such as Marlatt's relapse prevention model (Marlatt, 1985), also attend to "what's the matter" or the stuff that gets in the way for the patient. Such a model looks at these trouble spots as the cues that set off drinking.

Thus, when a patient complains, "We aren't talking enough about recovery and about AA," the therapist can help clarify the group's task by responding, "How would that help in terms of getting to know one another better?" or "How would that make it possible to understand more about the hurdles that are trouble spots for you in connecting to others and getting on with your lives?" The therapist might also inquire, "What if we talked about 'recovery' all the time, or even most of time in here, would that be helpful?" If the group (or the leader) takes too literally the mandate of the "recovery" group, it ties his hands in terms of maximizing the group's potential to do what a therapy group is best at.

The same kind of confusion may manifest itself in a similar way in groups for collaterals, where the only thing that group members want to talk about is their substance-abusing relative, thereby preventing group members from really getting to know one another (or themselves). Thus, the leader might say to such patients, "How do you think it will help us move along with the things that you want to work on if we keep talking about your family member?" "How are you going to come to know one another and to understand your own issues and how you work if we keep focusing on your significant other?" The leader's questions keep reminding members of the task to be accomplished and the potential of the group.

The Substance Abuser Who Wants to Leave Group "To Work on Her ACOA Issues"

With the increasing emphasis in the substance-abuse field on "working on one's ACOA issues," a patient sometimes raises the possibility of embracing an alternative therapy so that she can work on her "adult-child issues." An example of this recently came up in a group that I supervise.

> A member, who had been in a long-term substance-abuse recovery group for 2 years, one day suddenly announced that she needed to switch to an ACOA group. The group leader was understandably baffled. The recovery group had been in existence for several years and was working at the level of a well-formed therapy group. Family-of-origin issues, as would be expected in any well-functioning psychodynamic therapy group, were part of the fabric of group life. Although ACOA issues were clearly important for this member, her proposal to leave the group in order to work on them puzzled the leader.

This issue challenged the leader to reconsider the purpose of the recovery group. If it was, indeed, a therapy group, why wouldn't family-of-origin issues be relevant? And if the family-of-origin issues were not seen as appropriate for a recovery group (if people had to leave the group in order to work on them), what would happen to those members of the group who were not "fortunate enough" to have parents who were alcoholic (i.e., people whose parents were, perhaps, dysfunctional in some other way)? What would these group members "graduate to" to work on their family-of-origin issues? In fact, long-term recovery groups generally involve less and less supportive activity and more family-of-origin work as the group evolves. In this context, it makes little sense to siphon off members (often those who have moved the farthest along in terms of understanding themselves) into separate groups to deal with their ACOA issues.

When this comes up in a group it may be helpful for leaders to inquire, "What issues do you feel you would deal with in an ACOA group that you are unable to deal with in here?" If the patient mentions some particular issues, the leader might inquire further about why the patient feels that those issues would not be appropriate for this group. He might also explore whether, in fact, such issues had been dealt with in this group already and wonder about the patient's current feeling that "somewhere else" would be a more appropriate place to deal with them.

It should be noted that sometimes a wish to leave the group in order to go on to an ACOA group may not reflect eagerness to explore issues in greater depth, but the opposite. It may reflect a wish to externalize one's problems by focusing on the alcoholic parent—safer territory when self-exploration begins to feel frightening. In addition, in changing to a new group, the momentum gained in the previous group is frequently slowed down. Thus, the move to another group can aid resistance—helping the patient to avoid doing what she may fear (while, of course, on the surface giving lip service to the opposite).

Conceptualizing Therapy: Trying to Determine What the Questions Are

Often we find our patients pushing us to "provide answers." The job of the therapist is to try to figure out what the relevant questions are behind this push for answers—and what the shared task is that she and the patient can meaningfully pursue to further the patient's growth. Thus, when a patient asks a question, the therapist's task is to try to determine, "What is the question to which my answer would actually be responding?" Often our patients are making much simpler assumptions than we are about the nature of their exchanges with us. For example, the patient says, "I just want to know whether or not you are recovering," but we assume that his question asks for more. We assume that he wants to know whether we can help him, whether we will understand, whether his needs will be adequately met. In a sense, throughout the therapeutic enterprise, we frequently take the patient (and his questions) more seriously than the patient may take himself. We assume that there is often more in human interactions (and in the patient's interaction with us) than initially meets the eye. If all were, in fact, as simple as it might seem on the surface, human emotions and interactions would not be so confusing, nor would they lead to the kinds of complications in our patient's lives (and in our own) that we often see. Although the patient says, "I ask a simple question and I want a simple answer," we know that often there are no simple answers and, also, that frequently the questions themselves are rather complicated.

Although imparting this message can sometimes lead to a feeling that the patient and therapist are now at loggerheads (the patient just wants a simple answer, and the therapist seems to be withholding), nonproductive stalemates can often be avoided if the patient understands that the therapist is taking him very seriously, even if he is not at this moment responding in the way that the patient would like. The therapist's message should be, I take you very seriously, and, indeed, I think an important question is being asked here. I would like to understand more about the question. Thus, the therapist might say (particularly to a patient who keeps repetitiously asking for a response to the same kind of question), "You know, I think that there is something very important that you want from me, and I think there is something real important going on between us. Do you think it might be helpful if we could better understand what that is?" The therapist might also say that he would like to give the question a little more thought because, indeed, he does feel that something important is happening here.

Even if the patient is disenchanted with the strategy that we are employing, it is important that he understand that our responses are meant neither to be flip nor to be dismissive. The therapist might even say, "You know, I could give you a quick response to that question, but I am not so very sure that would be helpful." Most of our patients have gotten answers that were all too quick most of their lives—free advice, easy solutions, and quick cliches from teachers, parents, and others telling them, "What you need to do is . . .." And these kinds of quick answers (which the patient often seems to be wanting from us when he asks, "Why can't you just tell me what to do?") are usually ineffective and all too often ignored. The therapist may say, "I understand that you feel it would be helpful if I just gave you a quick answer, but I'm not sure how useful that would be. My guess is not very. Probably lots of people have told you all kinds of quick things about your drinking—'Just stop,' 'Just go to meetings,' 'Find something else to do when you feel bad,' etc. All of us have gotten lots of advice, and all of us know how to rebuff it, as well."

Although I do not tell my patients what to do and rarely give advice, my questions often uncover options that the patient has never considered, or, if considered, has rejected out of hand. My questions also explore his resistance to considering options that would make his life more manageable. My goal is to remove the roadblocks so that he can freely make choices and expand his array of options, rather than giving him advice about any particular option that "seems best."

Integrating Past and Present

The task of therapy is to help patients integrate past and present to form a continuous fabric—to pull together split-off parts of themselves and pictures that do not seem to connect.

> *A group member repeatedly described his past and all the characters in it (particularly his mother) as bad. In contrast, the present was described in a benign way with all characters "nice," "good," etc., with "no problems or conflicts." His presentation in group was, in fact, so extreme that when he described incident after incident of horrible examples from his past (e.g., when his mother drowned one of his kittens), the group would respond unempathically—trying to introduce balance by saying things such as, "You have to understand that our parents had problems too," or, "It's not fair to see your parents in such a totally negative light."*
>
> *The therapist, wishing to help this patient integrate his simplistic, split-off views of past and present, good and bad parts, conceptualized the situation as follows. In the transference the patient acted only on the*

positive "mother" feelings—hanging on to the therapist's every word and letting her know that much of what she offered was useful. She suspected that some of these positive feelings belonged in the past (to his mother and other caregivers). Moreover, she assumed that the revulsive negative feelings that he described from the past were also alive (though well hidden) in his present relationships. In other words, it was her guess that the positive feelings that he was playing out with her also belonged, in part, to his relationship with his mother, and that some part of the negative feelings that he attached to his mother were also likely to be experienced with her (the therapist).

Thus, she decided that the next time he shared a revulsive story, she would ask whether there was anything like that going on in the group. More specifically, when he shared his next horrific cat tale, she asked, "Was there any piece of what you've been sharing that feels familiar in here?" To this the patient responded, "Of course not, we don't have any cats in here!" To this the therapist responded, "Well, I wasn't thinking so much of the cats, but of some of the feelings about your mom from back then that you still carry with you. You had a lot of powerful feelings toward your mom when that was going on, and I wondered whether you might be aware of some of those feelings coming up just a little bit in here?" The therapist's questions suggested that she would expect feelings from the past to resurface in the group. She then said to the patient, "One of the ways that therapy works is that small pieces of feelings from the past get reawakened in the therapy group, providing an opportunity to understand these important feelings and work them through in a new way. It wouldn't be surprising if some of these feelings come up, perhaps in small doses, toward me or toward other members of the group—in fact, it is just what we would expect."

Since the patient also talked about his present life only in glowing terms, the therapist also began inquiring, "If there were some parts that weren't going quite so well, do you feel you would be able to talk about them in here?" In addition, she said to the patient, "Sometimes when you talk about how things were and how they are now, I get the picture that what you experience is that the past, and all the characters in your past, were bad and that you were too; and that now, all of the characters in the cast, yourself included, are all good. My guess is that, with time, both the past and the present will appear more mixed, as we understand things better in here." That, of course, is the goal of therapy—to integrate the unconnected, split-off views of oneself including those that have become compartmentalized into "me in the past" versus "me in the present," or "me with some people" versus "me with others." The seeds of the good feelings that we carry into the present come from the past, and the residue of the bad feelings from the past remains with us in the present.

Viewing Therapy as a Journey in Which "Curiosity" Is the Guide

Therapy is a journey that the patient and therapist share, in which there is a quest for knowledge and an attempt to explore and investigate new paths together. Since the therapist does not want to go on such a journey with a patient who keeps her eyes closed, the therapist's task is to enlist the patient to *look around* with him. Thus, the therapist's task is to get the patient curious and interested in looking for clues and signs along the way. The therapist may encourage this by asking questions such as, "Are you curious about that?" If the patient says "No," the therapist might ask, "How come?" or, "Ever wondered about why you weren't curious about this kind of thing, given that it happens so often and seems to get you into such fixes?" Or the therapist might ask, "Is it curious to you that you haven't been at all curious about it?"

Alternatively, the therapist may raise the patient's curiosity about a long-held belief, framing it as a "notion"—implying that this idea may not be as factual as the patient might have believed. In other words, the therapist may translate a "fact" that has the quality of being a dead-end, nonnegotiable issue into a "notion" worthy of exploration. Thus, the therapist might ask, "Where did you get the notion that . . . ?"

Promoting Self-Evaluation

A self-reflective stance in the patient is facilitated by a therapist who helps the patient to evaluate for herself both what is going on and what it may mean. As Kanfer and Schefft (1988) clearly state, the therapist's role is to help "the client to evaluate and make value judgments but (he) does not do it for her" (p. 102). Accordingly, they advise therapists to guide the client so that evaluations about a situation or any conclusions about an action and its consequences are generated by the client and not the therapist. Because many people find it difficult to rely on their own internal evaluations, both about how they feel and how they are doing, an important leader task is to promote self-evaluation. Thus, it is helpful for leaders to make interventions that will help the patient to assess for herself how she is doing and the progress that she is making.

For example, a patient who feels that his presentation to others is always incompetent and bumbling might be asked at the end of a group session in which he has expressed himself well and has connected to other members, "Bob, how do you feel about your participation in the group this evening?" Leaders might further ask Bob how he felt about how he presented himself to others and how he felt about the responses that he got back. Other members might also be asked to give their impression of Bob's involvement in the group that evening. Often, this is a more useful and, in the long run, more change-promoting intervention than a more direct leader appraisal such as, "You seem to be coming across very clearly tonight, Bob."

Another example might be a patient who has been avoiding discussion of an important issue (e.g., a patient who will be having a divorce hearing in 2 weeks and has known about it for a while but has not been processing it in the group). The therapist might be tempted to ask the patient why she hadn't been talking about her upcoming hearing. It might be more productive instead to comment, "I wonder if you have had any thoughts, Diane, about the fact that you're going to be having your divorce hearing in a couple of weeks but haven't been talking about it in here." Whereas a "why" question may lead the patient to feel defensive, as if she somehow has to rationalize her failure to communicate, the latter question, we would hope, would help the patient to take a more self-reflective stance. The message that we would want the patient to have is that we are interested in her thoughts about what has gotten in the way. It is the obstacles that are important and interesting for us to take a look at. For example, we might say, "Diane, you're going to court in two weeks and have barely mentioned it. Have you wondered at all about what's been going on that has prevented you from bringing it up in the group?"

Encouraging patients to be able to judge for themselves how they are doing and the progress that they are making is also useful with regard to interventions about outside-of-group successes. As therapists, understandably, we are often very proud of our patients when they succeed. (Sometimes we even view this as a way of measuring our own success.) The patient's knowledge that her therapist is proud of her is by no means information that must be "hidden" from the patient; however, it should not be the primary focus. It is the patient's feelings that are important and should remain so—not the therapist's.

It is also important to remember that events that are *outwardly* unambiguous "successes" may be perceived ambivalently by the pa-

tient. A therapist who jumps in too hastily to compliment or con-
gratulate may miss an important opportunity to explore the meaning
of an event with the patient. Let us take, for example, a 40-year-old
woman who has been living at home with her elderly alcoholic parents—unable to separate and move on with her own life. After months
of debating about leaving home and searching for an apartment, she
decided to leave, and has taken a lease on an apartment at some
distance from her parents' home. The therapist might be inclined to
respond enthusiastically with something like, "Mary that's wonderful!" However, a more cautious and potentially more productive comment might be, "How does it feel to see yourself having gotten to this
point?" Or the therapist might start out with a comment such as, "It
must feel good to have been able to take this step." (Even here the
language is in terms of how it feels to the patient rather than to the
therapist.) This might be followed up with an inquiry about additional
feelings that the patient may have had. It is important for us to remember that even successes may not be unambivalently joyful experiences. Patients may feel anxious about the fact that things will be
different and worried about the loss of what has become familiar. They
may also be fearful of failure, or fearful that supports that have been
available when they were not doing so well may vanish now that they
are moving ahead. It is important that the therapist leave room for this
kind of exploration.

This chapter has attempted to capture some of the broad landmarks
that characterize the journey of the dynamically oriented interactional
therapy group. In the chapters that follow, roadblocks that impede the
journey are addressed as they manifest themselves in the group as a
whole, in individual members, and in the group leaders.

❖ 7 ❖
Removing the Roadblocks in the Group

The well-prepared leader will not only have a clear idea of what the journey will entail—what to pay attention to and how to get there—but will also be adept at maneuvering around the inevitable roadblocks that may hamper movement in a forward direction. Such roadblocks are frequently referred to in the psychotherapy literature as forms of resistance—defenses that are erected to avoid doing work that may be painful. Such roadblocks slow down the journey, or temporarily create an impasse that impedes progress. The next three chapters look at roadblocks that occur in the group as a whole, in individual members of the group, and in the group leaders themselves—providing, in addition, techniques for maneuvering around the roadblocks or removing them.

It should be noted that the line differentiating group, member, and leader roadblocks is not always clear, since they often interact. Sometimes what appears to be a member roadblock may actually be a roadblock for the group as a whole, in which the group allows a single member to represent or "contain" some piece of resistance that is shared by other group members. Thus, for example, a member's failure to pay his bill or repeated lateness may start out as a resistance in that individual member. Yet, if it continues and the group as a whole fails to take it up, it is very likely that this individual is enacting something for the entire group (otherwise the group would not allow it to continue). With this caveat about the potential overlap among the three categories of roadblocks, we begin with those roadblocks that are the most clearly localized in the group as a whole.

It may be helpful to think of the group's defensive activities as falling into three major categories:

1. *Distraction activities.* The group actively engages in one topic or issue as a way of avoiding a more important one, by focusing on outside-of-group crises, by joking around, or by engaging in patterned interactions.
2. *Avoidance defenses.* The group ignores painful material by acting as if it does not know what is going on, by behaving unempathically, by clamming up (use of silence), by ignoring important self-disclosures, and by using other forms of flight.
3. *Displacement.* The group talks in a displaced way about the therapy group—for example, when the group talks about how much they hate their weekly meetings at work or particular AA/Al-Anon meetings.

GROUP DISTRACTION ACTIVITIES

Topical Distractions

Often group discussion, though ostensibly important and seemingly relevant, is in fact serving as a defense against other more painful material. When the group seems to be eagerly engaged in a topic but the leader feels somewhat disengaged and uninterested, this kind of distraction or defensive maneuver may be operating. One variation of this was discussed in Chapter 5 in which the group uses the group theme defensively—focusing on alcohol/drug talk or talk about their chemically dependent relatives. Even if the leader has no idea what the group is defending against, once she tunes in to the fact that something is missing in the exchange, it is her job to help the group uncover what is not being talked about.

The following vignette provides another illustration of this kind of distraction activity:

In one group, following a very intense session in which aspects of a sexualized transference were heatedly discussed, the next session began (and continued for nearly 45 minutes) with members happily chatting about their outside lives—sharing delightful tales of two of the members' new babies, another member's grandchild, and other "updates" from their lives outside the group. When the leader asked members halfway through the session to examine the territory they had covered during the first half of the group, she was told, "It's been a long time since we've had a chance to check in with one another about our outside lives, and we needed some time to catch up." They went on to talk about how nice it was to get these updates and to be in touch with other aspects of one another.

The therapist can often dislodge the group from its defensive activity by taking the following steps: (1) making observations (or asking patients to do so) about what has been transpiring; (2) exploring feelings about the observations; and (3) connecting the observations and feelings to present and past group process. Thus, when the group seems stuck, even if the leader herself is confused about what is going on, it is useful to begin by asking for group members' observations. I might say, for example, "We're halfway through the meeting at this point; where have we been so far?" or, "What observations have people made about what we've been doing in here for the past 20 minutes?" I might then follow this with a question about how people feel about what we have been doing. Even when the group begins by defending (usually a bit lamely) what has been going on as "just fine," exploration of group members' feelings often helps to give the group leader a clue to what is happening.

The third step involves a hypothesis or interpretation that the leader puts out that may help the group to better understand what is happening. But even if the leader has no idea about what is going on and is not in a position yet to make any kind of formulation, she may enlist the group in solving the mystery. For example, the leader might say, "Though it seems like the group has enjoyed having a chance to 'catch up' and to find out more about what's been going on for various members in their home lives, it's unusual for this group to spend so much time focused outside the group. How might the amount of time we have spent on this be related to what went on inside the group during our last session?" In the example above, group members slowly began to recall the heated discussion from the week before and acknowledged that perhaps it was "too hot" in the group and that the time spent discussing outside things helped to "cool things down."

I find that even when I have no recollection of what went on during the prior group that might have caused the current resistance, the group members inevitably provide the missing link—responding with something like, "Oh, you mean the stuff about how we feel about the therapist?" or, "You mean the fight that Bob and Jenny were having?" Once the group is engaged in this process, it is dislodged from the stuck position and is able, once again, to move forward.

Outside-of-Group Crises

Outside-of-group crises may also be used to distract the group from doing the here-and-now processing of perhaps *even more difficult* issues within the group. Thus, the patient who presents with one crisis after another from her outside life, while getting the group engaged, also gets it away from exploring potentially conflictual within-group issues. It is useful to note that this kind of "distraction activity" may also be used as a defense mechanism in patients' outside lives as a way of managing and distracting themselves from conflict. For example, patients often create chaos in their lives and then complain in therapy about the disarray that they are experiencing. It is often helpful for them to understand that, despite the discomfort of the chaos, this chaos may serve a "distracting" function that keeps them from being in touch with other even more uncomfortable parts of themselves. This distraction can take many forms: taking on too many commitments, creating or precipitating battles at work or with family members, procrastinating to a point where disaster is imminent, etc. But often these self-imposed crises serve the same function—to "distract" against something else that would be even more difficult to look at.

Group Laughter as a Distraction

Although laughter can provide a sense of joy and movement to the group, at times it may also serve a defensive function. When the latter appears to be occurring, it may be useful to help group members understand that the laughter may be a way of avoiding painful material. Leaders may say something like the following: "The laughter that is occurring in here right now may be a way of dealing with some of the very difficult things that people have been sharing this evening." Even if the group does not immediately redirect itself to the more difficult material at hand, a comment such as this underscores for the group the seriousness of the issue at hand and the ways in which painful material can be avoided. It also underscores to the individuals whose issues were being processed that they are, indeed, to be taken seriously.

Repetitive, Patterned Interactions

Patterned, repetitive interactions between two or more members may similarly serve a group defensive function. Exchanges of the following variety often serve as a defense against change: "You started it!" "No, you did!" or "I can't stand it when you do X!" "Well I wouldn't do X if you wouldn't do Y." When two or more members in the group get engaged in one of these tightly cyclical and recursive loops, a situation is created in which there is total predictability. Even if the pattern is experienced by all participants as "negative," it protects participating members and the group as a whole from the even more frightening work of moving on and tackling weightier issues. Leaders can often interrupt these recursive loops by asking the participants questions such as the following: "John, did you know what Sally was likely to say when you said X?" "Sally, did you know what John was likely to say when you said Y?" Since both participants are likely to answer, "Yes, of course," the therapist would then inquire what use it might serve for them to engage in this dialogue when the expected outcome is so apparent to both of them (as well as to other members of the group). This kind of distraction activity or defensive maneuver should come to signal to group members that something important is being avoided. It is the leader's task to help the group figure out what that might be and then to move on.

The Group That Demands More Structure

When a group is having difficulty tolerating the emergence of increased intimacy, members will often propose to the leader (or even demand) a different kind of group format—usually one with "more structure." This is particularly likely after the first few weeks of the group and, later on, at turning points following increased self-disclosure among members. At such points, the leader may be prevailed upon to try something different—more didactic material, more structure (e.g., role plays), or some other way of formating and structuring the group. When the request comes up, it is helpful for the group leader to explore what the group hopes will be accomplished by the change in format. For example:

> *In one psychodynamically oriented group the members decided that it would be a good idea for the leader to provide more structure by doing role plays. This request for structure came several months into the group following several sessions in which members had become more intensely involved with one another on an emotional level, which for many felt quite frightening. The request for more structure was thus a way of controlling the intensity of the emotional life of the group and providing a sense of greater safety. (Of course, none of this was articulated by the group and, for the most part, was initially out of their awareness.) The group leader handled the request by asking, "How would it help to have role plays in here?" "What would the group accomplish that it is not accomplishing now, and how would things be different?"*
>
> *To each response the group made, the leader then would ask, "Is there some reason that we could not get to that particular material the way we are doing it now?" or, "What do you suppose gets in the way of our doing this in the format we now have?" Ultimately, she suggested to the group that there might be some connection between the recent increase in emotional intensity and the group's request to alter the format. She asked, "Do you suppose there could be a connection between what has been going on in the group the last few weeks—particularly the fact that members have been encountering one another more directly and sharing more personal material and the group's request for a change that would structure things more?" The leader was thus helping the group to understand that its request for change reflected anxiety in the group about the headway they were making and the greater intensity that was emerging and was a way of slowing things down. (Even the discussion about it served as a temporary detour.) She underscored this point by asking the main protagonist, "Do you think that you and Bill would feel more engaged with one another if Bill were playing his father and you were playing his mother, or do you think that you would feel more intensely engaged with one another if you were directly encountering one another, as you did in the session 2 weeks ago?"*

It is important to recognize that whenever a group moves forward there is also an inclination to take a few steps back. Temporarily tying the hands of the leader by making her feel inadequate is an effective maneuver, since a leader who is feeling this way is less likely to push the group to work. In the wake of feeling criticized by a group that is suggesting an alternative format, it is easy for the leader, as well as the group, to lose track of the fact that the group may, in fact, be making considerable headway and performing very effectively. It is important that the leader help the group keep track of its progress, even in the wake of a defensive maneuver that may temporarily belie that progress.

GROUP AVOIDANCE ACTIVITIES

The Group Knows but Won't Say

Often information is available to the group—at least unconsciously—that has not been directly dealt with. The group operates as if by not acknowledging what they know they can pretend that it is not so, and thereby avoid dealing with it. This kind of defense can often be effectively undermined by bringing in the information as an already-known fact that has been available to the group all along. Thus, for example, in a group that has never commented upon the therapist's pregnancy—now well into its eighth month—group leaders might begin addressing the issue by assuming that the group already knows about it. This can be done by simply asking, in relation to almost any group content, "How does this relate to my being pregnant?" or "How does this connect to the fact that I will soon be having a baby?" Similarly, when a group has long ignored the tremendous weight fluctuation of one of its members, the group leaders might ask (again in connection with even the most minimally related material), "How might this relate to Martha's having lost so much weight in the last few weeks?" The group leaders might further ask, "What do you make of the group's not having noticed, or at least not having verbalized what they did notice (e.g., Martha's weight loss, other people's weight gains, a member's lateness, therapist's big tummy)?"

The Group Acts Dumb: We Don't Know Your Pain

Occasionally group members protest defensively that they can't empathize with a particular group member because they have not personally experienced the exact situation. For example, in one group, when a patient described in detail her mother's death, several members protested that they couldn't empathize because nobody so close to them had died; or in another group, when a member had been sexually abused by her father, the group made a similar protest. Such protests have to be understood as defensive maneuvers and a wish not to get in touch with the pain in all of us that resonates with pain in other people. As therapists, we understand the pain of our patients, not because we have experienced each identical painful situation that they have been through, but because we are in touch with the reservoir of pain in our own lives. We would be in pretty bad shape (and probably too disabled to work effectively) if we had to experience the precise, painful incident of every patient that we ever worked with. Rather, we understand our patients' pain because we have all had pain—we have all had losses, we have all felt our self-images shattered at one time or another, we have all felt bad, we have all felt violated in some way. These are the basic feelings of the human condition, and that is how we understand our patients, regardless of whether or not we have experienced the same identical event.

Just as we as therapists understand our patients' pain—through resonation with the reservoir of pain in our own lives—group members are able to resonate with one another's pain in similar ways. Our task is to help group members not close off or fend against connecting to one another's pain. Thus, when a member protests, "I can't empathize with that because it hasn't happened to me," it usually means that he is finding it too painful to tune in. I might respond with something like, "Do you think you're having trouble connecting to these feelings because they are not familiar enough or because, perhaps, they are all too familiar?" To this, if the patient responds, "But I haven't been sexually abused; nothing like that ever happened to me!" I might say, "Yes, I hear that, but my hunch is that in some other ways that are perhaps very important to you, you have had some experiences that would help you to understand what Mary is going through. Who hasn't?" I might also suggest to the group, "Sometimes it's harder to listen to things that seem familiar in some significant ways or to things that we do connect to (but would rather not) than to other kinds of material that is less sensitive for us. I wonder if that is part of what is happening right now. When you cut Mary off, perhaps it is also a way of cutting off pain that is all too familiar that you would prefer not to have to experience right now."

The Unempathic Response

Sometimes the group responds unempathically—even somewhat critically—to a member who is having a great deal of trouble. For example, in one group, a family member who was still very much enmeshed with her substance-abusing partner would let the group know what a hard time she was having. Other members, who also lived with substance abusers who were periodically "active," would repeatedly respond with slightly superior and unsupportive responses, such as, "I used to do that, too—you just have to let go." Or, "I can't stand the fact that you remain so stuck, Sally. Week after week you just sit there and don't make any progress!"

It is frequently the case when someone is being treated harshly by the group, being scapegoated or responded to in a less than compassionate way, that the recipient is representing a disowned part of other members of the group (particularly the member who leads the pack in the attack). It is as if the group is saying, "This is something that we despise—it is something we know a great deal about, and we would feel much more comfortable if we could see this particular thing as totally residing within her." There is thus a pull in the group to see the unpleasant characteristic as one that belongs solely to one targeted individual. That one person (or one seat in the room) contains it all, and if we simply deal with that person (or boot her out), we can get rid of this objectionable part of ourselves, as well.

The leader might respond to this group dynamic by addressing initially the unempathic members who lead the attack, suggesting, "It must be hard for you to hear Sally doing this stuff. I wonder if it might bring back memories of yourself that are quite uncomfortable to think about—things about yourself that you like to think are in the past and gone but may not be 100% behind you." Alternatively, if a lot of group time is spent focusing on a particular unpleasant characteristic in one group member (particularly if it feels as if the group is beating a dead horse), the leader might suggest, "The group has spent a long time dealing with Sally's 'stuckness' (criticalness, withholdingness, etc.). My guess is that part of the reason the group is so focused on this is that it's something everybody in here knows a little about and that this issue has a lot of meaning for the group. Perhaps the group is trying to kick this characteristic down and beat it out because it's too close to home and simply cannot be ignored."

The Silent Treatment

Group avoidance of difficult material may also be expressed through silence. The silent response may be given when extremely painful material is shared by a member for the first time and other group members are unanimously protecting themselves from getting in touch with what it stirs up in each of them. Alternatively, the withholding silence (also known as the silent treatment) may be used to express anger at a particular member or the leader. Silences that need attention—defensive silences—are very different from the "connected silences" in which group members are quietly in touch with their feelings. Connected silences are rich moments in the group that usually feel good. The leader's own judgment of how he is feeling during the silence is often the best guide to understanding what kind of silence it is—unless he is having trouble tolerating, for example, his own sadness during a shared silent moment. Connected silences usually require little intervention other than a gentle nudge to see if the depth of feeling can be heightened. Thus, for example, the leader may softly inquire if members can share a bit about what was going on for them in the silence, or might simply comment, "This seems to be a feeling that everyone in here knows a good bit about."

Tense or abortive silences, on the other hand, need active attention by the leader. While it is important that the leader not be too hasty in dealing with such silences (as a means of dealing with his own discomfort), it is also important that he not let the silence build so long that he begins to feel that there is an insurmountable tension in the room that he himself may not be able to break into. (One little barometer that I use is the first time that I feel myself swallow. I have learned from past experience, that if I let a silence go on much beyond this point, I find it more and more difficult to let myself in.) Such tense silences can profitably be addressed by commenting on the silence, exploring it, or paying attention to the silence itself as a group response that needs to be understood. For example, the group's silence after a member's lengthy and detailed account of an outside-of-group event can be examined by the leader's inquiring, "What's been happening during this silence?" Or, "What was going on for each of you as Jim was talking?" If group members have tuned out (which is especially likely if Jim is inclined to disconnect from others and to have them, in turn, disconnect from him whenever he speaks), the group's lack of response can be understood as a response in its own right that can help shed light on Jim's interactions with the group.

Group anger at the leader that is expressed through silence is often more difficult to cut through. The leader might say, "What has been going on just now?" Or, may suggest, "My hunch is that during the silence each of you has been having your own thoughts and feelings, and that it might be helpful if we could understand more about what was going on for each of you." If there is no answer, he might say further, "I wonder how we can understand people's reticence to speak up just now." If the group responds with further silence, the leader might comment, "I wonder what we can make of the fact that people come together to do something with one another and to connect in some way, and yet group members seem right now to be trying very hard not to connect. How can we understand this?"

It is important to understand that silence is a response. Particularly when the leader senses that the silences are withholding and angry, it is important to process them (as we would any other kind of resistance). Thus, we may say to the group, "It's important for us to understand what's being communicated by not speaking right now. Since in the last couple of minutes I've asked a couple of questions about the silence and nobody has responded, I wonder if the silent response is a response to me. Perhaps people are trying to tell me something in their silence, but I can only guess what that is. I need your words to understand it more fully."

If the group seems to be waiting the therapist out in a sort of withholding silence, the leader might finally say, "What would the group have me do? Should I join you and sit silently too? Does that feel like it would be useful?" In my experience, when the leader suggests the possibility of ending the struggle by disengaging, even temporarily, patients do rally. After all, they have invested something in coming to treatment—some part of them that wants something and that wants to get better.

When the Group Ignores an Important Self-Disclosure

Occasionally a group member shares something that is very important to him and over which he feels extremely vulnerable, and the group responds by simply moving on. Frequently, when this occurs, the member who has just shared feels too vulnerable to refocus the group, fearing that others have found it difficult to accept what he has shared (or, even worse, find it difficult to accept him). What is often the case, instead, is that members are uncomfortable about what they have heard (for example, a disclosure that suggests that a member is gay) and may not want to "hear" what they believe has just been said. As a result, they may flee from the material rather than questioning the disclosure further—projecting that the person who has shared it is "too uncomfortable" to proceed further with the material. If the group does move away from this kind of sensitive material, it is important that the leader refocus the discussion on the group process. Thus, the leader might say, "What happened just then?" or, "How did people respond to what Sam just shared?" To the response, "Well, I guess we didn't say much," I might ask, "What do you think that was about?" Or, I might address Sam directly, asking how he felt about the group's response while he was sharing a few minutes earlier.

My questions help the group to continue to talk about the interaction that has just transpired. It is very important, when the leader notices something important that has not happened, that she take action in the same way she would if an overt mishap occurred in the group. One of the important roles of the leader is to keep track of what is going on in the group, and if the group cannot handle the material, it is essential that the leader help the group not only to process what it is that they are bypassing but to understand more about the dynamics involved in the bypass.

The Group Moves into a Problem-Solving Mode

The group can also avoid difficult or painful material by getting busily involved in trying to "solve" one another's problems. Members may get actively engaged in giving advice, even competing with one another to find the best solution, as a way of avoiding sitting with painful feelings of helplessness that are being aroused in the group.

Often the group's move into an advice-giving mode follows an active solicitation for "help" by an in-need member—a request that is often doomed to fail. For most of us "good advice" is far too available. Often, in fact, the problem is not in knowing what to do, but rather, having the wherewithal to implement it. (Most of us also know how to ignore even the best of advice.) Thus, when a patient seems to be soliciting advice or the group moves into an advice-giving mode, it might be helpful for the therapist to intervene by commenting, "There seems to be a lot of pressure in here to get the problem solved. How would it be for you if we did not give you any specific advice, but just listened and tried to really understand how things are for you and how it feels?" This suggests that part of the work of the therapy is understanding—getting into someone else's head and trying to experience the world from his framework. The leader might then also encourage other members to share some of their own feelings and reactions, particularly feelings that resonate with issues similar to those of the member who has sought the advice.

The leader's questions help the group to understand that an alternative task for the group is to understand what is going on rather than to fix it. The leader might further say to the group, "You know, one of the things that is often most missing in people's lives is somebody who will really listen and really share in trying to understand what is going on." Helping people to better understand their inner experiences and how they relate to the world is the task of psychotherapy. We don't necessarily solve our patient's problems. Often the best we can do is to better understand what the problem is.

The leader, trying to help the group understand its task and the way the group works, may have to undercut certain assumptions the members have about what they think is supposed to happen in the group: that one member talks until another member (or the leader) stops it, as in an AA meeting; that the purpose of the meeting is to socialize; or that the purpose of the meeting is primarily to get advice and feedback (to be told what to do). It is important to intercept each of these erroneous assumptions. More specifically, to the group that remains fixated about getting advice, the leader might say, "It seems that many members in here believe that the best we can get from this group is advice. I have a hunch that we can do a lot better than that. In my experience people often give advice without even listening adequately to the problem. And maybe what we can learn how to do better in here is to really listen and to really understand what is going on for one another, even if we can't necessarily solve it."

The Group That Engages and Pulls Back

Occasionally a patient bravely puts out that she is disappointed with the group and needs to have more group time and attention. The group responds initially by getting engaged and subsequently by pulling back. This is illustrated by the following case example.

A patient who was working on similar issues outside of the group (her disappointment with her husband), came in to report that she had taken some steps to let her husband know more about her needs (particularly sexually). The group spent a considerable amount of time talking with her about this, and she remained the focus for the entire session and about half of the following one. At that point the group's attention shifted. The third session the patient came in feeling rejected by the group and proclaiming that she felt that the members were angry at her—not only for asking more of her husband (just the reaction she would expect, particularly from the men) but also for asking for too much from them. Group members' protestations that they were not angry, but that they too wanted some of the attention for themselves, did little to appease her. The therapist cleverly helped to reintegrate the young woman into the group by suggesting to her (and to the group) that she had become the spokesperson for an important issue in the group— the wish to be able to get more and to take active steps to let people know what was needed. Thus, the leader said, "Nancy, in a sense, led the way for the group by focusing on wanting to get more, and engaging the group with her around how to do this. The group did get engaged with her around this and, in the process, each member also realized that he or she also wanted to be able to get more. The ensuing tension in the group was related to everyone's awareness of wanting more and concerns about how you get it, what happens when you ask for it, and whether there will be tension created when you do ask." Thus, the leader was suggesting that Nancy was the spokesperson for all group members in terms of their wishes to get more from one another in the group and, also, in their lives outside.

Group Defense against Greediness

Groups often develop mechanisms to defend against feared greed— the fear that other members will take too much, thereby thwarting each member's own forbidden wish to have it all. For example, one group member may take on the mantle of making sure that things get evenly divided in the group.

In one group, Miss Take would take an agenda at the beginning of each group and keep track of who had dealt with their material—making sure that the other 7 members had all completed their turns before she would speak. On the surface it looked as if this young woman—the bastion of group fairness—was concerned about making sure that everyone else was taken care of. But it is useful to ask what might have been going on for this individual, and for the group as a whole, that supported the recurrence of this task. To explore the issue, the leader asked, "What do you suppose would happen if you just started talking right at the beginning and didn't wait for the others to take their turns first—how much time do you think you would take?" To this, Miss Take responded, "Eleven and a half minutes, that would be my share." The leader then asked, "Can you imagine ever wanting to take more than your share?" This question was met with an adamant denial; "No, of course not—it would be greedy to take more than my fair amount!" The leader then asked, "Can you imagine that anybody else might ever want to have even a little bit more than his share?" To this, Miss Take responded, "Well, sure, I can imagine it." The leader replied, "You know, I can imagine that virtually everybody in this group at some point has wished that they could have more than their share—and perhaps even wished that they could take the entire session for themselves."

In the example above, Miss Take, by addressing this material in the same way every week, was actually speaking for an important issue in the group—all members' concerns about their greed. Patients will defend less against forbidden wishes if they understand that the wishes are just part of being human. All of us, at times, would like to have it all. (In fact, the wish is probably that we could have it all, all of the time.) Of course, since we are socialized beings, we give up acting on this wish because we have other needs that are also very important—particularly the need to be connected to other people. These two sets of needs compete; one cannot have it all and also be connected to others. But that does not mean that the wish itself is unacceptable. And it is important that group members come to understand this so that they don't have to defend so massively against these wishes when they do occur. Whatever group members, or the group collectively, are defending against is always more acceptable—once they come to understand that the feelings are quite normal and natural.

In this particular group this issue and its solution, the agenda, at times took on such importance that if the leader tried to help the group process what was going on in the group, the group became impatient—indicating that they felt that he was taking them off the track (that is, moving them away from "The Agenda"). This group had become so taken with their defensive strategies regarding allotment of time and covering the specified contents of the agenda that they had totally lost sight of the purpose of the group and the importance of group process. They acted, in fact, as if they were coming to a lecture and that a certain amount of material would have to get covered in each session.

In another eight-member group, the issue of group greed and "who is entitled to what" took an amusing turn when one of the quieter members claimed that she would be happy to have even less than her share, "just 20 minutes—or even less." To this another member, quick with his arithmetic, protested (only partly in jest), "Martha, you pig! There are eight of us in here! That's nearly twice your share!"

Group Resistance to New Blood

The arrival of new members in a group—especially when the group has been stable for a while and is beginning to feel cozy with the existing members—is a highly mixed and charged affair. Many members will have younger siblings and will remember (even if vaguely) the feelings of being displaced by the new arrival. Even in a small group where members have been requesting additions, mixed feelings are frequently plentiful when the arrivals actually come on the scene (just as children who beg their parents for a brother or sister are often less than enthused once the deed is actually done).

> In one group, the night that two new members arrived, the most recent member prior to their arrival interrupted the flow of group material by commenting, "I can't believe that we're talking about all this nonsense— who feels what about who, etc., etc., when what is really important right now is that Panama has been invaded." The leader commented, "It's understandable that major invasions would be on group members' minds tonight, since it has been some time since we took in even a single member let alone two at the same time. Tom's comment, I think, speaks to feelings that he as well as others in the group are feeling, about the integrity of the little nation that's in the room right now."

It is often helpful to begin addressing the conflictual feelings, whenever possible, before the newcomer actually arrives. This can be facilitated by coupling the announcement of the new arrival with questions to the group about the feelings raised by the announcement, how members imagine the newcomer will affect the group, and what they hope the new member will be like. I often ask, "What does the group think it needs right now?" or, "What kind of a person (age, sex, etc.) do you think the leader will choose, and why?"

One way of introducing the new member to the group is to invite him, as well as the "old-timers," to reflect upon what it is they are hoping to get out of the group, and for the older members to also talk about how much progress they feel they have made on the original goals that they set for themselves, as well as the work that remains. This process provides the dual opportunity for older members to set new goals and for newer members to gain hope by hearing the "veterans'" progress reports.

To empathically join the old members to the new members, the leader may ask the old members if they remember what it was like for them the first night they came in. Thus, I might say, "My guess is that each of you remembers pretty clearly your first night in the group and what was going on for you; can you share something about what that first night was like?" This helps the older members to empathically and sympathetically join with the new members, with comments such as, "Yeah, I was scared to death," or, "The first 5 minutes I was pretty sure I'd never come back." Or, an older member may recall, "I was afraid that nobody would like me—or that people in here would think that I was really nuts." The feelings that the older members share will resonate with what the new people are feeling and will help join them together. In this way the new members will know, not only that the old members understand what they are feeling, but also that the uncomfortable feelings are quite natural and, with time, pass. Or, an older member might say, "I just remember thinking, God, I hope somebody will talk to me, and worrying that I'd be ignored all night." The leader might then say, "Do you think that might be a little the way Jim (the new member) is feeling right now?" She might then turn to Jim and say, "Is that kind of the way you're feeling, Jim?" The leader has thus created a connection.

When a newcomer enters the group (regardless of whether it is a member or leader), it is also helpful to encourage the group to reflect upon how well they are doing at "welcoming" the new participant.

Thus, the leader might ask, near the end of the first session or perhaps during the second session, "How well is the group doing at welcoming Mr. New?" The group's reflections on how welcoming they have (or have not) been will not only make the new member feel more comfortable but will also explain, if inadequate welcoming has taken place, what this is about (thereby also helping the newcomer not to take personally the group's failure to welcome). The following case example will illustrate.

> *In one group, members gave an uncharacteristic "cold shoulder" to an incoming member. To the leader's question, "How is the group doing at welcoming Joe?" members responded, "I guess we're not," indicating that they too had noticed the chilly reception. The leader then asked, "What connection might there be between the group's behavior toward Joe and members' comments last week regarding 'the coziness of the group just as it is.'" With discussion it became apparent that the chilly response was directed more to the leader than to Joe. As one member put it, "We would have given a hard time to any new face that walked in—it's just too bad we took out our anger on you."*

To aid welcoming a newcomer, one of my favorite techniques is to ask the group to do something like a "group Rorschach"—a sort of projective technique in which the group is given an opportunity, in a very nonstructured way, to "describe itself" to the newcomer. Thus, the group may be asked, the first night a new leader comes in, what they think would be helpful for the new leader (or member) to know about how this particular group works. The leader might ask, "How does this group work?" or "What is this group like?" or perhaps, "How does this group function?" When this kind of question is asked, the newcomer learns about the group's perceptions about itself and how it functions, as well as the group's perceptions of "the rules around here." Group members commonly respond with remarks such as the following: "Well, for one thing, leaders rarely answer questions directly," or "We're mostly a pretty nice group—people are generally fairly gentle with one another" (perhaps a warning to the newcomer about how he is expected to behave). What the group chooses to share provides a handle on the members' perceptions of what the group is like and what it means to the members, and may also give clues about the expectations they have regarding how the newcomer ought to behave.

Changing "Time Zones"

In all dynamically oriented therapy (individual or group), there is continuous movement between present and past, and important work to be accomplished in both arenas. As group members explore present dysfunctional patterns that have repeatedly recurred in their lives, they will gain mastery as they understand how current patterns replicate childhood binds and outmoded solutions. While both past and present are important, each can also be used defensively to take flight from frightening work in the other arena. The following examples illustrate this kind of defensive activity:

> In an ACOA group, in the midst of an intense here-and-now focus in which two members were struggling to express their anger and competitive feelings toward one another, a third member interrupted to say, "I don't really see how Ted and Jane's dislike for one another has anything to do with the work that we're supposed to be doing here. I thought we came here to understand what our parents did to us." This protest can be understood as a defense against fears of emotional overload and a wish to return to safer material.
>
> In another group, when one member began to talk for the first time about her relationship with her alcoholic father, she struggled through sobs to share painful memories that hinted of sexual abuse. Another member, whose traumatic history shared similar events, interrupted by saying, "You know, Carla, there is just so much you can accomplish by complaining about your parents. We have learned in here that we have to take responsibility for our own lives—regardless of what our folks did or didn't do when we were little."

In both instances, the group has used a seemingly legitimate group focus to defend against painful work. Since both past and present focuses are important and legitimate, it is the leaders' job to know when to help the group move toward one or the other. The group will be most alive and engaging if leaders help it to move toward greater affect—understanding movement away from feelings as a defense. At times, the leaders will simply interpret the group's defensive maneuvers by saying something like, "It seems as if Carla's memories about these painful times with her dad are hard for the group to stay with. It's a kind of pain that's very familiar to many people in here, and there may be a wish to push it away." At other times, when the leaders feel that the group can stay with the painful feelings, they may try to help the group get back to them. For example, leaders might encourage the group by asking, "What makes it difficult to stay with the feelings?" or, "What thoughts or feelings were others having as Carla talked about her situation with her father?" Clearly, there is a delicate balance between the present and the past, and times when the group defenses will simply be noted, as opposed to other times when the leaders will push for greater exploration.

Differential Time Zone Resistance in ACOA versus Relatives Groups

Although any group can become temporarily stuck in either past or present, ACOA and family members groups have peculiar defensive forces in this regard (as described in Chapter 5). More specifically, in ACOA groups, members are more inclined to focus on the past— appropriately, as when they are dealing in a useful way with family-of-origin issues, or as is often the case, defensively, when the past is used as a way of avoiding important here-and-now interpersonal issues. In contrast, in family members groups, members often become riveted to (that is, defensively focused on) the current traumas of the chemically dependent people in their lives. These group members are often less comfortable working on family-of-origin issues and often, initially, may also be somewhat harder to engage in a here-and-now process focus within the group. These groups often require more shaping and help by the leaders to deal with either the historical antecedents or the "here-and-now" process.

DISPLACEMENT

Discussions of Other Groups as a Displaced Way of Talking about the Therapy Group

Up to now, we have been talking about group defensive operations that are used to help the group avoid certain painful material. Another kind of defensive activity involves talking about the relevant material, but in a camouflaged way. For example, the group may spend time talking about groups that they find troublesome. There may be complaints about staff meetings at work, where "nothing ever seems to get accomplished" or "people who don't seem to take their work seriously." Particularly when other group members also seem to be actively engaged, it is important to consider the possibility that the group is actually talking about itself in a displaced way. In groups with substance abusers, ACOAs, and other family members, it is particularly common for this kind of group displacement to occur around discussions of AA, Al-Anon, particular step meetings, etc. Common complaints include, "The meetings are too long and boring"; "Sometimes people come intoxicated"; "The speaker went on and on"; "It feels lonely, I don't feel connected at these meetings"; etc. Although discussions about any outside group should be a signal to the leader that the group may be talking about itself, special attention should be given to group talk that focuses on how uncomfortable it can be to be in a group with other substance abusers or their family members and all the things that may be disturbing about this. Thus, whenever 12-step groups are being discussed in the therapy group, and particularly when there seems to be some group energy around this, leaders should ask themselves whether members may be talking about the therapy group.

This chapter has focused on the roadblocks that occur within the group as a whole as the group attempts to slow down its journey or to block forward motion through the use of distraction, avoidance, and displacement activities. The next chapter examines roadblocks that serve some of the same functions for individual members of the group.

❖ 8 ❖
Removing the Roadblocks within the Patient

For every patient there is a conflict between doing the task that he comes to do and the resistances that oppose it. Even the most highly motivated patient, who comes to therapy wishing to change certain things about himself, has a life history and character structure that is built around being exactly the way he is. The forces of resistance can be extremely powerful.

Other patients come to us with even more mixed feelings about the therapy venture that they have signed up for. Although there is some motivation to get help (sometimes more external then we might wish), there may also be a sizable part of the patient that has serious reservations about engaging in the therapeutic work. The "good patient" is one who embraces our view of the treatment process and the treatment contract (at least by his outward behavior). But even such "good patients" may have their share of ambivalence, which may emerge as the work goes on. Our task is to maintain the alliance in these patients as resistances emerge, and to create an alliance, as well, with the patient whose ambivalence is more obvious from the start.*
It is important that we encourage patients to talk about their ambivalence and use these discussions to let them know that we understand the issues and will attempt to join with them despite (or even around) their ambivalence.

---

*In his discussion of substance abusers, Howard Shaffer describes these ambivalent patients as beginning the process of fighting their addiction with the "wish they could want to change, but [whose] ambivalence about their behavior may sabotage their efforts" (*Boston Herald*, November 7, 1989).

Initial ambivalence is often signaled in the group by the new member's focus on the differences between him and the other members. The patient may attend to demographic differences (age, marital status, employment status), drug of choice, or aspects of the course of his recovery—any of which can be used to "demonstrate" that "I am different, and my unique issues are not likely to be addressed." This kind of initial resistance can often be handled by helping the patient to see that each member of the group feels different in some way from all others, and each is, indeed, unique. Yet one thing that all members have in common is that they share this feeling that in some ways their situation is different and that they are unique.

This early indicator of ambivalence may resurface throughout the life of the group and is joined by many other forces of resistance as well. These forces of resistance—the hurdles in the patient that have to be overcome in order to achieve his therapeutic goals—are outlined in this chapter.

We begin by examining some of the more obvious indicators of resistance, expressed by group members' behavior when they deviate from the group contract. We then examine many other common patient hurdles that the group and the leader must overcome—forms of resistance that are broadly grouped into two categories: (1) withholding defenses and (2) disruptive defenses. Finally, we end the chapter by looking more generically at leader techniques that are helpful in providing a smoother journey for the group member.

DEVIATIONS FROM THE CONTRACT

The therapeutic contract sets a clear framework of expectations against which the deviations can be productively examined (see Vannicelli, 1989, for a fuller elaboration of this). The clearer the rules and expectations, the easier it is for the therapist to determine from the deviations what is problematic for a particular patient. The patient's deviations from the contract tell us about the nature of his ambivalence regarding the task that he came for—and more. We make the assumption that what is hard for the patient in terms of carrying out the group expectations is also hard in negotiating life outside the group. Thus, deviations from the group ground rules are useful in helping us to understand important aspects of the patient's dynamics.

The Patient Who Comes Late

Coming on time is the group ground rule around which deviations most commonly occur. Lateness may reflect ambivalence about coming to the group on a given night (or more generally) and may also provide a fertile opportunity to examine the ways in which group members deal with the commitments that they make. Thus, when a member comes late, I might first inquire how her lateness might relate to things that have been going on for her recently in the group (and her feelings about the group). If lateness is repeated, I might ask, "Is your coming late an expression of the way you handle commitments? Are you late to other things as well?" If the patient responds that, in fact, she is late for most things, I might say, "Well, perhaps you are bringing something to the group that gives us a chance to understand how you relate to lots of situations." Or if the patient says, "No, I'm only late to this" (an equally useful response), I might ask, "What is it about this?" Thus, the lateness is a piece of behavior which, in itself, can be profitably explored.

Addressing initial erosion of this ground rule can also be one of the most productive ways of helping group members to understand the commitment that they have made to one another and the seriousness of the task that they have embarked upon. The questions that leaders ask regarding lateness will help underscore why it is so very important to be on time. Since invariably something is going on in the group at the point that a member walks in late, I might ask the late member, "I wonder how it feels, Mary, to walk in knowing that John was in the middle of sharing something important and that you have missed a lot of it?" My question thus says very clearly that, when you walk in late, you're walking into the middle of something important. It is also useful to explore what the experience is like for the person who has been interrupted, by inquiring, "John, you were sharing something important, and I wonder how it felt not to have Mary here from the very beginning?" Of course that is what matters about the lateness— that a member was not involved in what was going on. The interrupted member is likely to respond, "Well, it did feel like sort of an interruption," or, "I don't feel like repeating it all."

If the leader asks questions in this way, the person who comes in late is bound to have some feelings about it. The questions that I ask embed statements that force the group to examine the issue and give members an opportunity to process together why it matters if people are on time. (It is not just that it is not nice, or that there is a rule about it, or that a social convention is being broken; it really matters for the effective functioning of the group.) I might also ask members if they thought the group might be different if they could count on one another each week for the entire session. Thus, I might ask, "What do you think it would be like if everybody were here and on time every week? How might that affect the way we work?"

The Patient Who Doesn't Come

A patient's decision to "skip a group" should never be taken lightly and needs to be explored. Often, even seemingly legitimate reasons for being away—"a cold," "important business engagement," etc., may add to ambivalence that is already present. While the surface explanation should always be taken seriously, the leader should not assume that this is necessarily the whole story. More blatant absences need even more active intervention. For example:

> In one group a member (Bob) failed to show up for a session during which one of the co-leaders was on vacation. When asked the next week what might have been going on for him, he responded, "I was tired, and it didn't seem that important to be here." When the now-returned leader wondered whether the feeling that "It didn't seem that important" might connect to her own absence the previous week, other members (also angry about her absence) tried to let Bob off the hook—responding, "The guy is doing well and felt like missing a week; why not?" The leader helped process this further by stating that perhaps there was some feeling that since she could be away when she was feeling OK, that perhaps members might be justified in doing the same thing. But she also wondered, "What do you think this group would be like if, when members were feeling OK, they just decided not to come?" The discussion helped to clarify the importance to all members of having the entire group present—and the loss and disruption that was felt when people were missing.

The Patient Who Owes the Group Money

It is not uncommon, particularly in clinics where the billing is handled by someone other than the group therapist, for some group members to run up large bills. Group leaders often feel, when member debts are brought to their attention, that this should be handled in some way "outside of the group"—in order not to "embarrass" delinquent members. However, precisely because money is such a hot topic, it is particularly productive for the leader to handle all transactions and discussions about money in the group itself. In our clinic, we have a specific ground rule indicating not only that patients need to be current with their payments but that if anything happens that makes it difficult to pay on time, these difficulties must be discussed in the group. Thus, the patient who is remiss about paying and has not discussed this is actually in double jeopardy.

It is important to remember that issues around money and payment have complex meaning for patients—particularly feelings that love and caring should not have to be paid for. (Often these feelings correspond to the therapists' own feelings about this—particularly when they themselves are not getting paid very much by the agency that they are working for.) However, when the billing and payment are brought directly into the room, there is an opportunity for many complicated feelings about money to be expressed and explored. Such complicated feelings are illustrated by the following examples.

> One young woman protested bitterly when her therapist placed the check in clear view on the table between them—proclaiming, "Can't you get that thing out of the way!" With exploration, it became clear that she wished not to be reminded of the financial aspect of their relationship, and of the accompanying feeling that if she did not pay, her therapist "wouldn't care two hoots" about her.
>
> In another group, one member acted out her rage at the therapist who she felt "neglected her" by periodic late payments ("forgetting" to bring in the money) and bounced checks. When she began to work in the group on her anger and disappointment with the leaders, the delinquent payments ceased. However, a few months later, she overpaid her monthly bill. When the leaders pointed this out, she commented with a laugh, "Maybe now I'll finally get credit!"

Money is often an especially loaded issue in clinics where members are charged differential fees based on income. As Yalom (1975) points out, the "privates" of the group these days have less to do with genitality and sexuality (which are often discussed with ease) than with the fee structure, "because often money and fees act as electrodes upon which much of the feeling toward the leader is condensed" (p. 199).

Thus, how much one pays is often one of the group's most tightly guarded secrets, "since differences in payment by the members (and the silent insidious corollary, differences in rights . . .) threaten the very cement of the group" (p. 199).

One way to introduce the issue of delinquent payment is to state that it has come to the leader's attention that some members are behind in their payments and to suggest that there is sometimes a relationship between nonwork in a therapy group and nonpayment —that is, that people who are not working in the group are also, frequently, the ones who are not paying. This correlation can go in two directions. If they aren't working in the group and they aren't getting much out it, they may not want to pay. On the other hand, if they are not paying, they may not feel that they deserve any group time to do their own work. Thus, the therapist might say something like, "Some of you who owe a lot of money haven't been doing a whole lot in here the last couple of months, and I wonder if there is some feeling that if you're not paying for the group that you aren't entitled to much of the group's time."

> In one group, leaders productively used the nonpayment/nonentitlement equation to suggest to the group that settling the group's debts would be necessary to provide a forum in which members could begin to really use the group's full potential. After months of chipping away at the issue of members' reluctance to fully utilize the group (with repeated updates also about the status of members' financial standing with the clinic), the group moved on to a higher level of intimacy and group development.

A perhaps unexpected sensitivity about money sometimes occurs in patients who have (or have had) a great deal of it. In extremely wealthy families, there is often a taboo around talking about money. For example:

> A young man whom I was treating had grown to be very self-conscious about his family's considerable financial status and felt that any allusions to money were extremely private. In the course of our pregroup interviews as we began negotiating the fee (his current situation was not so solvent, as he was supporting himself through law school), I asked him how much he and his wife were currently earning. He stuttered and stammered and turned bright red. When I asked what reaction he had to my question, he was extremely discomforted, stating, "I've never been asked such a direct question about money. We never talked about money

in my family—it's the kind of thing that we would never tell anybody."
As we discussed it further, it became clear that part of the complicated
feelings had to do with a sense that he had always had far more money
than he should, and that rich people carried a burden of shame that went
with their having too much more than others.

The Patient Who Catches the Therapist "On the Side"

Occasionally a group member will catch the therapist just after the
group—or as the group is exiting. Regardless of the content of the
communication, it is important that the therapist encourage the patient to bring the material back into the group. This can be done, first,
by keeping the therapist-patient interaction to a minimum in this
outside-of- group context and, second, by letting the patient know that
it is important that she bring up whatever has been shared between her
and the therapist during the next session. If the patient fails to bring
it up, it is the leader's task to do so. Rather than sharing the specific
content, however (this I would leave to the patient), I might bring it
up as follows: "Mary, after group last session you shared something
with me. Were you planning to bring it up tonight?" If the patient says
"No," this should be explored. The therapist might ask, "What
thoughts did you have about wanting me to know but not the group?"
Even if the patient discloses that the material is "too personal" to share
with the group at this point, it is useful for the group to know that
something important is going on with her and, also, that something is
going on either within her or within the group that is getting in the
way of her talking about it. Moreover, the therapist is reinforcing the
norm that outside-of-group communications will be brought back in.

Invoking the Group Contract

If a group member breaks a group ground rule, it is important to
remind the group of the rule and its importance—especially in the face
of the fact that it has just been broken. This might be done by saying
to the group, "How does the group feel about Karen's behavior, in
light of the ground rule that we have about this?"
   If a group member responds, after breaking a rule, that he is afraid
that the group is going to give him a hard time (e.g., the patient who

comes late, or the patient who meets with another group member outside of the group), the patient might be asked, "How would it feel if the group didn't give you a hard time—given that, in fact, we do have certain expectations in this regard?"

Fine Line between Feeling Protected and Feeling Controlled

Another way of thinking about the group therapy contract is that the guidelines and expectations, if adhered to, may help the patient to feel contained and protected—as if somebody else is "minding the store." Thus, for example, calling a patient on his lateness to group may be reassuring, since it gives the message that there is someone in charge who is going to make sure that things go well. On the other hand, there is a fine line between feeling that somebody is looking out for one's well-being and feeling controlled. While some patients may feel relieved that they are held accountable for behavior that deviates from expectations, others will feel that they are being controlled, over-protected, and patronized. It is important to look at both aspects of this conflict.

WITHHOLDING DEFENSES

The Silent Member

While silence in the group as a whole (particularly if prolonged) is hard to ignore, the individual member who is silent is often overlooked.* Yet, silence in an individual member, as in the group as a whole, is a "response" that needs to be examined. As therapists, we should assume that everything that the patient shows us about himself tells something about his strengths, as well as giving us a window on "what is the matter." In this light, the patient who is characteristically silent (noted for his nonresponse, refusal to share, etc.) should be viewed by the therapist as showing us a piece of himself that needs to be understood. The patient's response of nonresponding may give us a handle on difficulties he has connecting to others or, possibly, even difficulties staying in touch with himself.

---

*See Chapter 7 for a discussion of silence in the group as a whole.

The Patient Who Talks about His Feelings but Is Emotionally Distant

People can be out of touch when they are talking, just as when they are silent. Sometimes, in a show-and-tell fashion, a patient reports what is going on in his life outside of the group, along with a "commentary" on how he felt, which has a story-like quality devoid of real feeling. Although the therapist may be tempted to point out to such a patient that as he speaks the feelings seem to be lacking, or to say, "You don't seem at all angry," or "You don't seem sad," it may be more useful to gently help the patient to experience the unexpressed feeling. Thus, I might say, "Are you feeling any of that anger right now?" I would be asking him whether he is connected to any of those feelings currently, as a way of determining the extent to which he is allowing the feelings to actually register. Or, I might ask more questions about how anger feels—for example, "When you do start feeling angry, what happens for you?" Or, "How do you show that you're angry?" and "How do you show it in here?"

The leader's job is to try to help the patient with his problematic behavior (e.g., inability to connect to his feelings in a way the group can respond to) by slowly inching him toward more appropriate responses. Although sometimes it works to simply describe to the patient what is missing in his presentation (i.e., the feelings), often such observations simply heighten the patient's defensiveness and produce more of the same. Confrontations such as, "You're not telling me what you're feeling!" or "You're just intellectualizing!" often produce more of the same because the patient may not even be clear about how he could be doing it differently. It is often helpful if the group leader can walk around the back door a bit and coax him in, rather than simply telling him that what he is currently doing is not right.

The Member Who Keeps Others in the Dark

The group member who keeps others in the dark surprises the group with information "after the fact"—presenting major life changes after they have been accomplished, without ever having shared or processed them in the group. For example, the group barely knows that a member has been dating, and suddenly an engagement is announced; or a

2-month leave is suddenly announced as a fait accompli in order to take a class that the patient signed up for months earlier, without discussing it with the group.

In one group that I supervise a particularly graphic after-the-fact announcement occurred:

> *Mary, during her third year in the group, suddenly announced that she was 5 months pregnant. The group was baffled and enraged about how they could have been left in the dark for so long. Mary responded by protesting that she, herself, had only "recently learned of the pregnancy"—citing some confusion, "since I was on some pills that made it hard for me to understand whether I should be getting my period or not." The group leader, seeing this as an opportunity to help both the group and Mary understand something about Mary's dynamics, suggested that perhaps part of what the group was angry about, not only now but repeatedly during the course of Mary's group work, was that she frequently kept people in the dark (herself as well). Group members would often say to this patient, "Get real, lady!" or make other comments indicating that somehow there was something unauthentic about her communications. But what the therapist appropriately understood was that, at times, Mary not only was unreal with the group, but also had trouble being real with herself. As a result of keeping back important material, others often felt out of touch with her, as did she with herself.*

With such a patient it is useful to explore what her "out-of-touchness" is about. Is it that she doesn't notice things around her, or that she doesn't assign meaning to what she notices, or that she does notice and does assign meaning but just doesn't want to let other people know about it? It is important to learn more about where the block occurs. Is it intrapsychic, or is it interpersonal? Thus, with this patient the leader might have asked, "Did you know that there were changes happening in your body? What did you make of it? How did you decide not to do anything about the cues that you noticed? When did you start thinking that you might be pregnant?" With a patient like this, it is important to understand what blocks essential information from getting into the appropriate channels. Thus, it is important to ask as many questions as necessary to help get her in touch with internal cues about what might be happening—signals from her body, even fleeting sensations—that might help inform her about what is going on.

Another possibility with this particular patient is that ambivalence about the pregnancy might have contributed to her not paying attention to the cues. What was most striking, in this particular group, was that another member was also pregnant (and also in her fifth month) and had been talking about it for nearly 4 months. We might even wonder whether Mary's ambivalence made it harder for her to recognize the signs of pregnancy and made it even more difficult to raise it in the group. One of the most difficult topics for people to talk about—perhaps even more difficult than family incest or sexual abuse—is ambivalent feelings, or even downright negative feelings, about having a baby. It is not culturally acceptable to not want to have a baby who is living inside of you. One can well imagine, in particular, in this group, which had been oohing and aahing over another member's pregnancy for some months (a member who was delighted to be finally having a baby), what little forum Mary would have had for talking about ambivalent feelings that she might have.

In the group that we have been talking about, it should also be noted that by the time Mary was 5 months pregnant, she had looked quite heavy for some time. Several members volunteered after her announcement that they had actually suspected it. However, no one had asked. (The leader herself had been suspicious but had not said anything.) It was almost as if the group had joined the patient in her defense of not paying attention to what was going on. In such a situation it might have been useful for the group leader to say, "Mary, I wonder if in some way we joined you in something that is all too familiar to you—not noticing what is going on, or perhaps noticing, but not paying attention to it. Several people in here indicated that they were sort of aware that you might be pregnant. How would you have felt if somebody had asked you about it and paid attention?" In all likelihood, this young woman got messages early on that she should not pay attention to things that were going on around her, or even inside of her; and she lived that message out, developing a defensive style consistent with it. (In this instance, through projective identification,* every member of the group who had thought she was pregnant—and had ignored it—briefly joined her in the defense of not paying attention.)

---

*The concept of projective identification is more fully elaborated in Chapter 10.

The Patient Who Tunes Out

From time to time, we have patients in our groups who seem not to be paying attention—who look as if they are "spacing out." It is helpful to attend to such patients by tuning in to them when they seem to be tuning out. Thus, I might say to such a patient, "Where were you, Jim, as Sarah was talking?" If Jim responds, "Gee, I don't know; I think I just kind of tuned out," I might ask further, "Do you remember what the last thing was that Sarah was talking about before you tuned out?" This might help give clue to what in the material had been difficult for Jim to stay connected to. On the other hand, if Jim says, "I don't know, I was just thinking about my own stuff," it gives us a chance to hear more about what it is that is distracting him from being able to tune in and respond to others. Or, I might ask, "What do you think was going on inside of you while Sarah was talking that led you to tune out?" Our goal is to help the patient understand more about his tuning out—both within the group and outside of the group, as well. After commenting a few times on his spacing out, I might say, "It seems like when you space out in here, it's because there is something important going on that you are pulling back from. My guess is that you probably do this in situations outside the group as well, making it hard to stay feeling really connected to people. One of the goals of therapy would be to try to understand more about what it is that you feel you need to pull back from."

Our task is to help enjoin the patient to see his goal in terms of learning how better to connect to others. It is often helpful to tell patients, "A major task of therapy is to help you learn to connect better to yourself (what is going on inside of you) and to others. And when you tune out, you are showing us something about what is the matter with your connections—something we have a wonderful opportunity in the group to help you with." I might then ask, "Would it be helpful, Jim, when group members notice that you are pulling back, for them to give you that feedback?" If Jim agrees, I would then ask the group how they would feel about doing this. If the members were reluctant to agree—or agreed but later ignored his disconnections, the group's avoidance would itself become an issue (a group defense in the nature of those discussed in the previous chapter) and would need to be addressed as an indication that the group as a whole was avoiding issues around connectedness.

The Member Who Participates Only around the Issues of Others

Some group members, though actively engaged, rarely bring up material of their own. Such members often gain from the group experience by the feeling of connectedness to other people, as well as by learning to understand more about "how people tick." Much of this learning can take place (what people are about and how they are connected to one another) even during periods when a member is disclosing relatively little in terms of personal data about himself. The issues that he chooses to latch on to tend to be meaningful to himself as well; and through this route, he does an important part of the task that he is there for.

If the group leader, however, feels that he would like to encourage some members to participate more with regard to their own material, one technique that I like is to ask members how much they each feel that the group knows about them. (Sometimes I ask, more concretely, for percentages.) I might also ask other group members how much they feel they know about one another, and how much each member feels she would like others in the group ultimately to come to know. It is important to realize that there are no right or wrong answers to this—people differ tremendously in this regard. One member may feel that the group knows 50% about her and that she would be very happy if, ultimately, they came to know about 65% or 70%; another may feel that the group knows 50% but would not be satisfied until they came to know 90%. The answers are interesting and help us come to know more about another aspect of the individual—that is, how much he feels that he would like to be known.

This is also a very productive exercise in a couples group where I may say to each member of the couple, "How well does your spouse know you, do you think?" Then I might turn to the other spouse and say, "How much of you do you think that she knows?" I then might ask each of them how much they would hope the other would come to know about them, as well as how much they would hope that other group members would come to learn about them, both individually and as a couple.

The Patient Who Is Scared to Go On

Often patients present themselves as vulnerable and afraid of taking the next step, and they sometimes believe they are actually incapable of it. Although it is not appropriate to push patients to go farther than they are comfortable with, it is generally my experience that it is helpful to encourage them to go a little farther than they might believe they are capable of (and rarely, if ever, does such an invitation produce "too much" work). It is often helpful to give the reluctant patient the message, "You can pace yourself as you need to, but my hunch is that you can do more than you think you can right now." It is important to ally with the patient's strength and, while giving permission to pull back if needed, also provide the encouragement to go ahead. As Ann Alonso* says to patients at times of hesitancy, "This is something that you can talk more about—or not." She is thus giving patients permission not to go on if this is their preference, but also the message that they *can*. The message says, I think you can talk about this—it is certainly an option and I believe you can handle it, even though you might not think so; or, you can choose not to. Thus, in this short message, there is both an expression of confidence that the work can be done and also the option to choose not to if the patient does not feel ready.

The "Fragile Patient"

Often a patient's style of self-presentation in the group raises concern (both among members as well as the leader) about his vulnerability to confrontation. Such patients may present in a manner that suggests that if they get pushed too far, they may "break" or may flee from the group. The leader may also feel that she needs to protect such a patient, and may find herself doing so by deflecting rather than encouraging direct feedback and confrontation. However, it may be more effective for the leader to communicate that she wants to understand with the patient more about what is going on and what would be useful. Her questions are a way of psychologically moving to the patient's side and providing support. The message is, "I am on your side—I am in this with you." If the patient's response to an inquiry about what would help right now is, "I just want everyone to get off my case," the leader might say, "Well, let's understand how that might help. How would you feel, Jim, if every time you said something was

---

*Ann Alonso. Institute for Senior Group Therapists, American Group Psychotherapy Association Meeting, San Francisco, 1989.

tough, people just pulled away from you?" The leader might then say, "My guess is that it probably wouldn't feel so terrific, since often when people give messages to others to 'back off,' when others actually do this they feel somewhat abandoned—as if no one wants to have anything to do with them. How is it for you in other situations, when you give these 'leave-me-alone' messages?" I might further say to him, "People who give 'leave-me-alone' messages often end up feeling very lonely."

The Patient Who Fears Loss of Control

Often, in the initial phases of groups, fears about "opening up" may be accompanied by fantasies of being overwhelmed or of coming "unglued." The member who is feeling acute pain and is reluctant to get in touch with it may fear that if she gives word to the pain of her past, she may "cry forever." In this instance, the group leader might help the patient to articulate her concern while also gently challenging this idea. To the patient who responds, "If I start to open up, I might cry forever," the group leader might ask, "Did that ever happen?" Patients often respond with surprise to this question, since, of course, to some extent tears and sadness are always self-limiting. When the patient responds, "No, but I did cry for a long time," the therapist might ask, "How were you able to stop?" (thus focusing on the self-limiting mechanisms inherent in the patient). That one can learn ways of managing intense feelings, and that a situation that seems to feel a little out of control will not necessarily lead to total chaos and destruction, are important lessons for a group member who has lived in a dysfunctional family, where periods of being out of control frequently reached an intolerable level.

For some group members, the fear of "coming unglued" (associated, perhaps, with being hospitalized) may be a very real one. With such patients, the leaders can also focus on the patient's adaptive strengths while at the same time acknowledging the intense fears by saying something like, "I suspect that these fears of 'coming unglued' have been with you for a long time, and that alongside of these you've also developed ways of taking care of yourself. Perhaps at this moment you, as well as other group members, are having trouble remembering the ways in which you have been able to cope, even when stressed."

In groups in which members have greater psychopathology, other kinds of structuring and "cooling out" activities on the part of the leaders may also be useful to help lower a patients' fears about things getting "out of control" (for example, changing time zones to dilute intensity of affect, as discussed in Chapter 7).

The Patient Who Uses One Feeling to Avoid Another

Although many patients need help in expressing and differentiating the full range of feelings, including anger, many group leaders (and hence many members) stay focused on expressions of anger as an end in itself—disregarding the defensive aspects of anger. Although it is essential for many patients to learn how to recognize when they are feeling angry and to deal with anger appropriately, it is also important that both leaders and members understand that anger may be a defense protecting against feelings of vulnerability, weakness, and helplessness.*

It is important to note, in fact, that almost any feeling can be used defensively to avoid connecting with yet another that is even more painful. The following clinical example illustrates this kind of defensive activity:

> Following a particularly warm session in which a patient became acutely in touch with how much the group therapy (and the leader) meant to her, she came in the next week suspicious about whom the leader might be discussing her case with. The leader, noting the marked difference in tenor between the previous session and the current one (characterized by near-paranoid delusions about the therapist), commented, "As uncomfortable as these untrusting feelings about me might be, I wonder if perhaps they are more comfortable than some others that are even less comfortable." There was palpable relief when the patient smilingly acknowledged that this might be so, and began to talk about her increasing awareness of her tremendous attachment to the group and to the leader. As she put it, "Maybe we got a little too close for comfort last time."

---

*Allen Surkis takes the position that anger is always defensive—protecting against underlying fear of sustaining physical or psychological injury (at the extreme, physical or psychological death). Workshop: "The Group Therapist's Quandary—To Lead or to Treat?" Presented at 10th International Congress on Group Psychotherapy, Amsterdam, 1989.

For many patients anger tends to comes first, and only if the surface is scratched do the underlying feelings of sadness, vulnerability, and fear come through. For others anger may be more difficult to get to; such patients routinely respond with feelings of "hurt," without understanding that anger might also be present. Let us take, for example, a patient who reports feeling "really hurt," after being "called on the carpet" by his father in front of a friend. This response, while possibly reflecting some part of his feelings, in all likelihood also defends against the more unacceptable feelings of anger. The therapist, interested in exploring the full range of feeling, might say, "You were aware of feeling really hurt. What additional feelings came up?" If the patient is still unable to get in touch with his anger, the therapist might ask, "What do you imagine someone else might have felt in that situation?"

The case that follows illustrates successful use of this technique.

A group member was having tremendous difficulty getting in touch with his rage at finding his wife in their bed with another man—insisting for nearly 30 minutes that all he felt was "upset and hurt." When finally asked how he thought another man might feel had he just walked into his bedroom and found his bed occupied by another man, he responded, "People kill for that. You read about it in the newspapers all the time!" To this the leader responded, "So others might be angry enough to kill in that situation. Perhaps you feel that if you were to let yourself get in touch with your feelings you would be totally out of control."

Another strategy is also useful for helping a patient to get in touch with and eventually integrate unacceptable feelings of rage. The therapist can play back the "expectable" feelings, but with reduced intensity and in a manner that conveys that the feelings are understandable (and even "natural") under the circumstances. For example:

A patient who was repeatedly being imposed upon by his "always sweet" mother responded with passive aggression, while consistently disowning any conscious anger at her. When asked by the therapist, "Did you ever feel like telling mother off when these things happened?" the patient responded, "Oh no! My mother is so sweet and good, I'm sure that she has only my best interest at heart!" The therapist responded, "I can imagine that your mother's 'good intentions' might make it more difficult to say something to her if you do feel a little disappointed and irritated when she makes so many requests." (For some patients the word "irri-

tated" or "annoyed" heightens defensiveness less than the to-be-avoided at all costs word "angry.")

Another way of helping patients get in touch with their anger (while avoiding using the word angry) is to suggest that the patient might "be feeling a little sore."* This is a way of getting not only at the anger but also at the underlying feelings of vulnerability and rawness that usually accompany it. It's a gentle word that also has complex meaning and is usually comfortably accepted as a description of what is being felt.

The Patient Who Has Trouble with Sadness

As indicated above, patients who have trouble getting in touch with sadness may at times defend against this feeling with another that is more readily available—frequently anger. I might say to such a patient, "Sometimes people protect themselves from their sadness by feeling another feeling instead, such as anger. Are you aware of anything like that?" I might also suggest that for this member, anger might serve as a cue to the group that there might also be some sad feelings that we would want to try to pay attention to.

To help the patient inch toward sadness, I might also suggest, if I notice any slight change in the patient's facial expression, that the patient looks as if she might be feeling just a trace of that sadness right now. My inclination is to make it a small dose, particularly for patients who are afraid of becoming overwhelmed by their sadness. A small dose—just a trace—may be tolerable and may allow one to get closer to experiencing it. If the patient continues to defend, saying, "No, I wasn't aware of feeling sad," I might ask, "Do you think it is harder for you to let us know about the sadness, or to know about it for yourself?" This is an important question, because some patients are able to cry alone but not in the group; this is very different from the patient who is not able to cry at all. The patient who can cry alone, but does not allow herself to cry in group, may be protecting the group (or the leader) from her feelings or may fear being vulnerable in front of others. On the other hand, the patient who can't cry, even when alone,

---

*A lovely contribution from the late Norman Zinberg.

may fear that if she lets herself cry, the pain will be unbearable and she will never stop.

Other patients are aware that there is a feeling inside that they want to be in touch with but which they can't get out. The therapist wishing to help his patients get closer to feelings will avoid cognitive questions and try to ask questions that will inch the patient a little closer to the affect. Thus, to the patient who says, "I wish I could cry; I envy Mary her ability to experience the sadness about her father's death," I might ask, "How far away from feeling the sadness are you?" Or, I might ask, "Was there a time in here today when you felt a little closer to having that feeling?" If the answer is yes, I would ask the patient to share when that was and what she was experiencing— perhaps even sensations in her body that she may have been aware of at that point. I might also ask for memories or associations that she had at the moment of feeling a little closer to the feelings, some thought or feeling that might get her closer to the feeling that she was trying to get in touch with. Or, I might ask, "If you were to cry in here, do you have any idea what it might be about?" If the patient shares an event—such as "My mother's death"—I would ask for something in particular about it, some little thing that she finds especially sad as she thinks back. My approach is to help the patient inch her way into the feeling territory—looking all the while for signs that she is getting closer to the material, and, as I see her approaching this, helping out by saying, "I had a sense just then that perhaps you were aware of the sadness inside."

Or, I might say to the patient, "Your raising this suggests that there might be some of this sadness in you right now that you have a powerful wish to be in touch with. What would that be about?" After she discloses the general topic that she might want to feel sad about, I might ask, "What about that would you want to feel sad about? Are you aware of some little piece of that feeling even right now, as we talk?"

To the patient who seems reluctant about sharing sad feelings, I also might ask, "Did you notice that I had a Kleenex box on the desk?" and "Did you have any thoughts about what it might be for?" If the patient responds, "Well, I suppose some people cry in here," I might ask, "What do you think about that—do you think that it would be helpful for someone to feel that they would be able to cry in here if they were feeling sad?" The Kleenex box itself says something, and pointing out the Kleenex box underscores it. Basically, what it says is that I expect that tears are a part of expressing one's feelings and that this is quite to be expected in doing the work of therapy.

In a group, the value of crying can also be underscored by pointing out, the first time somebody does cry, that they have given a gift to the group—that sharing feelings helps the group to do its work. The therapist can also make it more acceptable in other ways, for example, by asking, "How does it feel to have been able to get so in touch with your feelings today?" "I wonder what it was like for others in the group that Carol was able to get in touch with these feelings just now?" The leader is thus saying, indirectly, let's pay attention to the fact that something important has happened here that is positive for the person who has shared and for other group members as well.

The Patient Who Tells the Group Something Is Going on That He Doesn't Wish to Share

The patient who lets the group know that there is something important going on that he cannot talk about raises, for the entire group, the issue of what can and cannot be shared and concerns, familiar to all patients, about the sanctity of their self-disclosures. This person, in a sense, is a spokesperson for the thorniest manifestation of resistance—namely, important things that are not being discussed. Often the group's inclination is to struggle with this individual to share (usually with little success)—a struggle that represents a wish to settle the ambivalence that resides in each member about how open he will be with the group. The leader may be able to use the reticent patient's sharing about his reluctance as an opportunity to examine more generally issues of safety in the group and each individual's conflicts about self-disclosure.

I might begin by addressing the reluctant member as follows, "It's clear, Bob, that you wanted us to know that there is something important going on for you—even though at this point you're not sure you feel ready to tell us what that is." I might then ask, "Do you have any thoughts about what it is about the group that makes you feel as if it would be hard to share this part of yourself?" I might then ask a few other questions such as whether this is a part of him that has been shared anywhere else and how he imagines it might feel to be comfortable enough with the group to be able to let them in on this part of himself. Sometimes the patient who shares that there is something important going on that he is not yet ready to talk about is almost ready, and this discussion may help him to open up. If not, other group members may soon become frustrated and confrontational—as Bob becomes the representation of everything that is withholding and protected in the group (and in each of them).

To make the issue more available to the group as a whole, I might then comment, "I have a hunch that nearly everyone in here has some part of himself that he has not yet been able to share with the group— something that he still feels needs to be protected." I would then explore group members' perceptions of what holds each of them back—both qualities of the group and their own issues. While I would not press for sharing of the actual content of the withheld material, such discussions often make it easier for such sharing to take place, and often some of the less-protected material will begin to be shared.

Looked at in this way, the patient who announces that he is withholding something offers a pearl to the group—an opportunity to focus on those parts of each group member that feel in need of pro- tection and, also, on the ways that the group operates that make it feel not yet safe enough. It gives group members an opportunity to ex- amine what they are there for and the group's potential to provide it.

The Patient Who Is Sitting on Something Awful from the Past

Sometimes a group member lets us know that something awful has happened in the past that she is reluctant to talk about. When some- one says, "I have a secret—something awful has gone on that I can't tell the group about," I am less concerned about the content of the secret than I am about the feeling that something horrible has gone on that cannot be talked about. To help a group member talk about this material, I might say, "Well, perhaps you are not ready to talk about the particular event just yet" (this often helps to relax the individual and says that we are not going to push), "but what do you think the group would come to learn about you if you did share what it is that you are feeling you need to keep secret?" I might also ask, "What do you think would happen if you did share it?" or, "What would it be like to share something like that in here?" Once the group member shares what it is that she fears that the group will come to find out about her—for example, that she is an awful person, the kind of person that bad things happen to because she is so very bad—she might not have shared the contents of the particular event, but she has, in fact, indicated the most important part of the secret (the shame about those parts of herself that she feels she must keep hidden). Generally in the processing of an exchange of this sort, one usually does come to hear about the event. However, the event itself and the particular details are less important than her fears about how people will feel about her if they know.

What matters most is getting past the initial fear that there might be things about oneself that can not be shared. Once one realizes that the group can contain the feelings (because some part of the traumatic event has been shared), then the individual is free to share more details (or not) as she feels comfortable. As one group member put it, "What is important is the knowledge that I could share—in fact that I could share every single detail if I wanted to, and I would still be accepted; moreover, that I have a choice about whether I will share any particular detail or not." (Knowing that it is possible to talk about something—even if one does not go into all the details—is often a tremendous relief, particularly when one has guarded a secret for a considerable amount of time.)

Whether one details the events or not, knowing that the traumatic event took place becomes an important part of understanding many aspects of an individual's interpersonal life, both within and outside of the group. The important dynamics and issues can be worked on without necessarily telling and retelling specific details. The issue is there all the time and will come up for the group member in many different ways as she comes to understand her relationships in the group.

Often group leaders experience a sense of pressure when somebody begins to tell his story. A feeling may be generated that a certain amount of the actual content needs to be shared. But what, exactly, needs to be communicated? For example, does it matter with a sexually abused client what specifically the sexual acts were, or where specifically they took place, or how many times? Any one of these facts may be important to a given individual to reveal, but none of them is necessarily essential to understanding the person's sense of being violated and all of the bad feelings that go with that. Often when there is a traumatizing event or series of events in a family, what is most difficult for the individual involved is the fact that it happened and, often along with this, a feeling that she is bad because it happened to her. In addition, the person involved is likely to have many feelings about growing up in the kind of family that this kind of thing could happen in and feelings about not being adequately protected as a child—in essence, basic human feelings that are understandable independent of any particular details.

It is important for group leaders to remember that we are not journalists trying to get the "whole story" or FBI agents trying to thoroughly investigate a crime, uncovering some singularly important fact. Clearly, the particular facts are not nearly as important as the many feelings that accompany them.

Anxiety and Resistance Following an Important Self-Disclosure

Often, after a patient has made an important self-disclosure in a group, this is followed by considerable anxiety: "Does this mean that I have to keep talking about it? Does this mean that if new people come into the group, I have to tell them too?" It is important that two messages are available to the patient after such a self-disclosure. First, "People disclose in here when they are ready," and second, "Now that you've shared this secret, you know that you can do it." The following case example illustrates the patient's dilemma and the manner in which it was effectively handled.

> Pat had begun to hint, by the end of his second year in the group, that there was something important that he had not talked about. Finally, he shared with the group that he was gay. The next week, as another older member was talking about his pending termination, Pat became worried about new members joining the group and expressed concern about whether he would again have to share his secret. To this the group leader responded, "You have been with us for 2 years now. What have you learned about whether people have to share their secrets and how soon?" (Obviously, this patient has learned that one can go 2 years without sharing a secret.) But the rest of her message to the patient was, "While you've learned that people don't talk about things in here until they are ready, you have also learned that you can now talk about this if you wish. That you were able last week to take the risk of sharing means that this option is now available to you."

This kind of concern is often raised in groups when new members are about to come in—older members asking, "Does this mean we're going have to go all the way back to the beginning, and I'm going to have to tell my whole story all over again?" But of course, we never go back to the beginning because group members are not in the same place they were when they joined the group. The group leader needs to challenge this kind of notion by asking, "How so? Are you in the same place that you were 2 years ago or 4 years ago?" To this, the patient will respond, "Well no," and the leader should comment, "So how could you introduce yourself now as if you were 'at the beginning'?" In fact, we never go back to the beginning. When new group members enter, they enter with members at their current stage of development. And similarly, the patient who has made his self-disclosure is also not going "back to the beginning" because he is now, also, in a different place. This can be suggested to the patient by saying, "Perhaps the fact that you have opened up the secret a little bit suggests that you are not feeling that it is so important to hide it any more. My guess is that this, itself, will have some bearing on how you conduct yourself with new members who come into the group."

The Patient Who Becomes Stressed When Recapitulating the Family Drama

Often patients experience a high degree of emotionality when they find themselves reliving, in the group, a situation that is just like an uncomfortable situation from their family of origin. Thus, the patient may exclaim, "This is just like it was in my own family, I can't stand it!" Often such patients are on the verge of prematurely and precipitously departing from the group—as the feelings are all too familiar. When this happens, it may be helpful for the group leader to point out, "You know, that's just what we would expect to happen in the group; you are giving us an opportunity to work on something that's real important, since what's happening now is something that's come up for you in significant ways before. I have a hunch this may be a turning point in your work—since you've allowed the group in, in a way that makes it possible for old themes to be recreated and for us to have a chance together to look at it. Turning points are always scary in therapy, but they are also real opportunities to move ahead."

The Patient Who Both Invites Closeness and Rebuffs It

Struggles around intimacy are a central theme in any therapy group (and probably in most therapy). The patient who most crisply articulates the group's conflict in this area is the one who both invites closeness and rebuffs it (sometimes sequentially and sometimes even simultaneously). Thus, like a puppy who barks ferociously and at the same time wags its tail, this individual is constantly expressing both sides of the conflict. Those who interact with her mixed messages are often unclear as to which message to respond to. Such patients, themselves, often feel confused about what they want. Perhaps what is best understood, if the therapist and the group are to fully empathize with the conflict, is that both messages express true (albeit conflicting) feelings. There is a real wish to invite closeness and to engage, yet at the same time there is fear and a sense of danger.

> In one group, a member repeatedly demonstrated this conflict as she would say (with a big grin) "all men are scumbags." The male members would be confused; was she playing, or was she hostilely rebuffing them? (Clearly, both.) Similarly, whenever a member attempted to get close to her by praising her work in the group, her style as a person, etc., she would respond in a hostile tone, "I don't know what you're talking about" or "I don't see how you can say that; last week you were saying that you objected to my behavior."

When Overt Content Contradicts Underlying Meaning

Often patients' protestations—particularly around issues of intimacy and closeness with the therapist—speak one message in terms of the overt content, while another message is covertly played out in the patient's behavior. Thus, while simultaneously criticizing the therapist (and perhaps other group members) for not being close enough, warm enough, giving enough, etc., the demand quality of the protest serves to push them further away. If the therapist listens to the overt message, he may hear that he has disappointed the patient by being too cold and too distant. Yet, what may be missed in such interactions is that such protests often follow closely upon the heels of an incident in which the therapist or group members have gotten too close. The protestation covers the very real anxiety about the closeness. For example:

In one group a young woman, following an empathic response by her group leader, began complaining about the content of the therapist's intervention. Touched by the empathic intent of the therapist but discomforted by the intensity of her own yearnings to be close (as well as the feelings of closeness that emerged at that moment), she handled her discomfort by protesting that she did not like the words that the therapist had chosen and proceeded to struggle with her (thereby creating distance between her and the therapist for the next several weeks). The therapist, confused and not understanding what it was that she had done, tried to clarify her words—missing the fact that the patient's discomfort was not related to the content but to the process between him and the patient and to their emerging closeness.

In another group a young woman used her protests about the therapist's failure to hug her as a way of creating distance after a particularly intense group session in which she shared her tremendous love for the therapist—sputtering out, through tears, "I . . . only . . . wish . . . it's . . . so hard . . . if only my real . . . mother . . . could have been . . . like you." The therapist, also very moved, made an empathic comment indicating how hard she knew it was for the patient to share this, and the session ended. The next session the patient returned, ragefully protesting that she did not know how the therapist felt about her, that she "would have expected a hug—or at least to have the therapist touch her hair or her shoulder or something"—adding that now she was sure that the therapist "didn't care about her at all." Again the patient's words, while suggesting that she wanted more closeness, were contradicted by the rageful demanding nature of her request; and the entire communication served (in keeping with the unconscious intention) to reestablish a more comfortable distance.

The Patient Who Makes Faulty Generalizations from a Weekend Marathon

Occasionally group members go off for weekend marathon groups with the hope of getting in touch with material that they have been unable to work on in the group. The opportunity to share with others in a time-limited format, where the patient knows in advance that the intimacy will come to an end, provides a safety net for many patients that makes it possible for them to share. (This is analogous in some ways to the freedom that many people encounter in a "shipboard romance"—where one can allow himself to get close and to feel bonded and connected knowing that there is no danger of long-term engulfment or commitment.) The advantage of the "shipboard-romance therapy experience" is that the patient has an opportunity to experience himself in a way that he may not have been able to do otherwise and learns that there are things he can choose to share that he had not formerly thought he could. This can be a very positive learning experience. On the other hand, if the patient falsely generalizes from his experience that the only circumstance under which he can share has to do with some of the specifics of that situation—e.g., it has to be a weekend program, or structured exercises have to be used, or the therapist has to have a certain style—he prevents himself from taking away from the experience information that can be generalized to the long-term group (and to long-term relationships outside the group). The following clinical vignette illustrates this kind of patient roadblock.

A group member who had been feeling "stalled" for some time went away for a weekend institute. It turned out to be a very positive experience for him, and he was pleased about his ability to open up and share some of the material that he had been feeling was "stuck inside." Unfortunately, through false generalization of what had been positive in the experience, and not understanding his own concerns about sharing in a more long-term relationship, he returned from the weekend therapy encounter with a decision to leave both his individual therapy and his long-term therapy group "to find a more structured kind of therapy." (He had mistakenly attributed his success in the weekend institute to its structure, rather than to its brevity, and the added comfort this gave him, given his difficulties opening up in long-term relationships.) The plight of this particular man was perhaps aggravated even more by the fact that he had been pressured into marriage by his fiancee's announcement that she was pregnant and now, just a few weeks after the wedding, he was dealing with an extremely demanding wife (and mother-in-law). Feeling trapped by the two long-term commitments with women that he had just taken on, the prospect of jettisoning the relationships with the two therapists (also women) seemed appealing. The group leader helped him to understand his current weariness about long-term commitments and the added safety in something that felt structured and brief. She also helped him to understand that his wish to leave both the group and individual therapy at this point made sense in the context of his new commitments but had little to do with what he actually could or could not do in a therapy situation. Moreover, she let him know that the fact that he had been able to accomplish something in the short-term group was an indication of his ability to let people know him and the impor-

tance of extending this ability so that he could do it in long-term relation-ships as well, without feeling that he would be "taken over" by the other person.

DISRUPTIVE DEFENSES

The Verbally Abusive Patient

The patient who is verbally aggressive or abusive with others, if too intimidating for group members to appropriately respond to, may cast a pallor over the group. Group members may feel that it is too risky to respond, or may fear that if they express what they are feeling they will be next on the "hit list." It is the leader's job to help provide a safe environment in which such interactions can be productively processed and understood—not only by the attacking group member but, also, by the other members (who need to understand what is motivating their reluctance to respond). When such interactions take place, the group leader may begin by directing attention either to the other group members or to the one who has been verbally aggressive. A response to the group as a whole might be something like, "What was going on for people as John was talking just then?" If the group responds in a bland way, I might further say, "John has been pretty forthright with some of his feelings this evening. It seems as if others in here are having more difficulty right now sharing their feelings. Perhaps we can understand what it is about what John has shared or the way in which he shared it that makes it hard to respond." If John's directness is at least in part appropriate, this comment suggests to John that he has done something useful for the group but that the group is having trouble responding to it. It also may suggest, however, that there may be something about the way in which he has done it that may be problematic.

An alternative strategy would be to address John directly by asking how he hoped the other person would understand what he just shared, and whether he felt that what he communicated was going to get the kind of connection with the other person that he was hoping for. Sometimes group members really don't know how they come across, and such exchanges can help clarify important aspects of their interpersonal communication style. Thus, I might say, "John, how do you suppose Mary might be feeling just now about your response to her?" Or, I might ask John to empathically put himself in Mary's shoes, saying, "If you had just received the kind of feedback that you gave to Mary, how do you suppose you'd be feeling right now?" This gives the person who has gone on the attack an opportunity to examine his own behavior and to reflect upon its impact. It may also give the person who has been attacked an opportunity to talk more directly about how she perceives the interaction and to give others in the group an opportunity to discuss it, as well.

I might follow up by turning to Mary and asking, "What was going on for you just then as John was addressing you?" I might then ask John if he had any idea that that was how Mary would have responded. And I would follow this up by asking, "Do you have any thoughts about what in your communication may have led her to respond in this way?" If John says, "Well, I was pissed, and I told her I was—that's the kind of guy I am," I might ask, "How well does that work for you?" If John responds, "Fine! If people don't like it, they scram!" I might respond, "Well, I wonder if that's one of the things that you're hoping to learn more about in here—how when you're feeling vulnerable or upset, you can let people know what's going on without pushing them away." It is helpful if the leader can empathically address the aggressive person, helping him as well as the rest of the group to understand his vulnerability in a way that makes him more human and less frightening. The leader might further inquire, "Is it like you to come across in the way that you have been tonight?" When the patient responds, "Yea, sure, like I told you! That's the kind of guy I am!" the leader might comment, "I wonder if that's the kind of thing that's caused trouble for you—that when you're feeling uncomfortable or when somebody's set something off in you, it's hard for you to let that person know how you feel in a way that will allow the two of you to stay connected to one another." The leader is thus saying that it is appropriate to let people know how you feel, and that people can learn in the group how to do this in a way that doesn't push others away.

The Patient Who Goes On and On

It is important to remember that often our patients have no idea what appropriate group behavior is. Sometimes the patient who goes on and on—seemingly talking until somebody finally interrupts him, is doing what he thinks is expected. This behavior may seem to be totally consistent with what he has seen in AA meetings, where one person stands up and speaks. It may also be similar to what he does in his own individual therapy, where he speaks until he runs out of something to say or until the therapist asks a question and he begins to speak again. Understandably, our patients frequently have little idea about what is supposed to happen in a therapy group.

It is important that the questions that we ask help them to understand what the group process is about and what productive group behavior will consist of. Thus, to the man who continues to speak on and on, I might ask, "Bob, what are you hoping the group will come to learn about you from what you have been sharing?" Bob may look up blankly and say, "Huh, well nothing really. I didn't really have any particular thoughts about that." The leader might say, "Well, from what you're saying, Bob, it sounds as if you're not real sure what you are supposed to do in the group or what kind of participation would be most useful for you; others in here also weren't so sure in the beginning and were also confused about how to proceed." I might then turn to some of the older group members and say, "Maybe one of you who has been here a little longer could give Bob a sense about how the group works and also what this group, in particular, is like."

It is important to remember that our patients need educating about psychotherapy. Few of them have read books about it, and even those who are knowledgeable about it (e.g., those who are therapists themselves), often find themselves somewhat confused, in their own therapy, about what is going on. We must understand that our patients almost universally experience this confusion. (I, myself, began my own psychotherapy while a psychology intern and continued it for nearly 4 years. For much of the first 3 years, I think I was genuinely confused as to what psychotherapy was all about—or at least my psychotherapy.) We must remember that confusion is not uncommon, and that sometimes patients talk on and on because they do not know what else to do. They may actually be relieved to have somebody stop them.

The Patient Who Is Difficult to Stop

In one group, members complained week after week that one member (Carol) seemed to monopolize the group time. When the leader appropriately asked why the group thought that they let Carol do this, the group responded, "She's impossible to stop." At this point, I might have turned to Carol and said, "Carol, is that so—are you really impossible to stop?" and might have asked further, "What do you suppose it would take for the group to slow you down in order to interact with you in a way that feels more connected?" I might then say, "My hunch is, Carol, that when you go on and on, sometimes you don't feel quite connected either; we need to find a way for you to be able to share in here that will let you feel more connected to other members and they to you."

It is rare, indeed, that a patient is totally unstoppable. Rather, the group is often in collusion—allowing an "unstoppable" patient to filibuster in order to protect all members from doing the more frightening work of getting to know one another. I might pursue the group a little further by asking, "How do you mean, she's unstoppable?" If a member responds, "Well, I tried to interrupt, but she just kept talking," I might ask, "What do you suppose keeps you and other group members from telling Carol directly that she is keeping you out or that you are having a hard time getting a word in?" I might also ask Carol, "Were you aware that someone had tried to stop you just then?" If Carol says, "No, I really wasn't—I guess I missed it," I might ask, "What kind of feedback do you think it would take for you to know that people wanted you to stop? Do you think it would help if group members signaled you in some way?" Or, if Carol said she had been aware that people wanted her to stop, I would want to explore further the fact that she continued speaking despite this awareness. Or if Carol responds, "Yes, I was aware that she was trying to stop me, but it made me mad so I just ignored it," I might ask, "How do you think we should deal with this?" (This question would be to both Carol and the group collectively, since the group as a whole needs to decide on a strategy that will help them move forward.) I make the assumption in many of my interventions that people come to a therapy group, in large measure, to learn how to be more connected. And it is our task to help group members learn more about how to achieve this goal by examining the ways in which they disengage and disconnect.

When the monopolizing patient complains that there are too many people in the group and thus not enough time for her to speak, it is sometimes helpful to suggest that the patient seems to have the notion that she is going to get better by talking a lot. We understand from this that what she is hoping desperately for is to be understood. However, since the formula that she has come up with—using lots of words—has not worked, she needs to find another strategy that will be more effective—perhaps using fewer words. Many patients, aware that their familiar ways of connecting serve them poorly, try the same strategy, but more so (e.g., it hasn't worked when I talk for 10 minutes, so I'll try talking for 20 and even faster). What may be needed is a different strategy altogether. Thus, the leader might say, "I think we can all understand that what you really want is for someone to listen and to really hear you, and my guess is that you haven't yet figured out a way to do that. The formula that you have come up with is that if you use a lot of words, maybe somebody will hear something. But I have a hunch that that hasn't worked and that what you are desperately looking for is another strategy that will work better." The bottom line of what we all want is probably not so very complicated— it is to be listened to and understood, tasks for which therapy groups are admirably suited.

The Patient Who Interrupts

The interrupter, often a member new to the group, repeatedly breaks in, creating frustrating discontinuity in the flow of the group's interaction. Sometimes such interruptions will have no obvious connection to the material at hand; at other times, interruptions will be phrased as a connection, "Yes, I see what you mean, because in my situation . . ."—the patient using his flimsy connection as a jumping-off point for his own material. Often, when this happens, the member who has interrupted is responding to his own anxiety about being heard and, rather than carefully following what has been going on in the group, is impelled by his own anxiety to look for the first available opening, lest he not get an opportunity at all.

It is important that the group leader help the interrupter to understand the basis for his interruptive behavior and his concerns about not having his needs attended to. The leader may do this by commenting to the group, following such an interruption, "What just happened?" Group members may then describe that Mary was talking about such and such and then Jim started talking about something quite different. To this the group leader might respond, "What do you think that was about?" To this group members might respond, "Well, its clear that

Jim just couldn't wait to get in," or, "He just seems real anxious to get in right now." This gives the leader an opportunity to talk a little bit about how the group functions and to empathically comment on the interrupter's behavior. Thus, I might say, "You know, Jim, my hunch is that you don't know us well enough yet to be certain that the group will pay adequate attention to your issues; thus, at this point, you feel quite a lot of pressure to be heard and understood. My guess is that when other people are speaking you are often so distracted by your worries about this that it may even be hard to completely follow what is going on."

The Patient Who Runs out of the Group Session

The group member who flees from the room during the session is generally responding to uncomfortable feelings that are being stirred up, and she is also communicating her discomfort in a very visible way. It is important that the leaders understand more about what is going on for the particular individual and the impact of this fleeing behavior on the rest of the group. If the group does nothing to intervene, it is likely that the departing member is speaking for an impulse that is present in others in the group as well. It is often helpful if the group can examine what the basis for that impulse in the room might be. The leader might say, for example, "My guess is that many of you, in fact, have felt at one time or another this impulse to 'beat a hasty retreat.' Any thoughts about how we are as a group that might help us understand the flight feelings that are coming up for us just now?" The leader might then explore what group members might do to help one another talk about these feelings when they do come up—underscoring that no matter what is going on in the group (including impulses to flee), it is essential to the therapeutic work that the members remain in the room to talk about it.

However, if a member repeatedly flees, it is also necessary to reiterate the expectation that all members selected for the group are assumed to be capable of remaining in the room and talking about what is going on. If the member is uncertain about whether she can adhere to this requirement, this needs to be discussed both in the group and individually if necessary, and her continued membership in the group reevaluated.

THERAPIST TECHNIQUES

Just a Gentle Nudge

Throughout this chapter, as we have dealt with particular roadblocks within the patient, we have demonstrated strategies that the therapist may use to attend to the patient's defenses. We have talked about ways of helping the patient to understand his defenses and also demonstrated ways of gently maneuvering around them when necessary. Although frequently our task is to help analyze the defense, equally often the therapist needs to "disarm the defense" (tiptoeing in the back door). Some may argue that this does not respect the patient's defenses, but I would argue that by so doing we respect his strengths. As Surkis* points out, the role of the therapist is to help the patient see that his defenses are not necessary by gently disarming him so that he can put aside his arms and briefly experience himself without them.† To this end it is often useful to "pull" rather than "push." The leader needs to disarm—and even to be disarming. The therapist must ally with the resistant patient, enjoining him to give up the struggle by siding with him. When the patient says, "I don't have any problems," or "I don't want to be here," the therapist needs to mobilize the part of the patient that is there.

I find that often the most effective interventions are those that are small and subtle—light nudges that gently turn things around. For example, the patient who feels left out might say to the group leader, "You seem to really like Jane." To this the therapist might say, "Only Jane?" (thereby encouraging the patient to consider the possibility that the therapist might like others in the group as well—perhaps including the protesting patient). Or, when only one side of an ambivalent message is expressed, Alonso** uses a technique that I particularly

---

*Allen Surkis. "The Group Therapist's Quandary: To Lead or to Treat?" Workshop presented at 10th International Congress on Group Psychotherapy, Amsterdam, 1989.
†Miller (1983), writing about motivational interviewing with problem drinkers, addresses this same issue, citing Goethe: "If you treat an individual as he is, he will stay as he is, but if you treat him as if he were what he ought to be and could be, he will become what he ought to be and could be."
**Institute for Senior Group Therapists, American Group Psychotherapy Association Meeting, San Francisco, 1989.

like. For example, a patient might say, "I certainly don't want to take all the time of the group." To this the therapist might gently respond, "On the one hand," suggesting that that might be part of how the patient feels, but that the opposite feeling—the feeling of wanting to take all of the group's time—might exist simultaneously. As a rule, the lightest, smallest intervention that will do the trick should be used. Of course, it takes skill and practice to know just how little may be needed.

On the Use of Shortcuts

It is often helpful to develop a shorthand expression with the patient that will capture an important part of her dynamics. For example, we talked earlier in this chapter about a conflict that the therapist (and group) came to refer to as the "barking tail." These shorthand expressions, particularly if they reflect a compassionate understanding of the patient's dynamics, make it easier for the group and the leader to refer to something that is transpiring without going into elaborate details.

Picking a "loaded" word can also be a shortcut to helping members understand an important dynamic that is being played out. Words such as "interloper," "illicit," etc. can help the group get in touch with powerful feelings. For example:

> An angry group member repeatedly used the excuse "I forgot!"—as week after week went by and he neglected to bring in his payment. The leader suggested that "I forgot" was the old "F-word," leading the group to talk about how such passive-aggressive maneuvers can be skillfully used to give the message, "Fuck you."
>
> In another group, the word "illicit" was applied to the activity of two group members who secretly met outside the group for a one-day hike. (It should be noted that one of these group members had been incestuously involved with his sister—also against the family rules.) The word "illicit" stirred up recollections from the past and helped this patient get in touch with a piece of the dynamic that he was replaying from his family of origin.

Questions that Embed Important Statements

It is often important to challenge incorrect beliefs that are held by group members. I find that questions are generally more helpful than direct statements in refuting falsely held beliefs—especially when dealing with misbeliefs about the status of the therapeutic relationship or the patient's sense of how the therapist feels about him. For example, in the midst of a negative reaction to the therapist in which the patient has felt injuriously challenged, the patient may blurt out, "Nobody has ever been on my side except perhaps Dr. X (the other co-therapist)." Rather than saying to the patient, "Oh, but I am on your side!" (a refutation which, at that point, would merely sound defensive or as if it were disputing unempathically the true feelings of the patient) I might say instead, "Is it hard to imagine that I am on your side?"

In a similar vein, to a patient who is hanging on to the false belief that she is an unattractive, ugly duckling, a simple refutation from the therapist would, in all likelihood, again be seen as unempathic. While the therapist might be tempted to say to such a patient, "But you are attractive," a more useful intervention might be to ask "What keeps you, do you suppose, from seeing how attractive you are?" This question gets at the heart of the matter—the patient's own defensive issues that lead her to see things other than as they are. They are not simply statements of refutation by the therapist, but rather, encouragement to examine more about the process.

Another example of this, when patients want to confirm that the therapist cares, can similarly be dealt with. The patient might taunt, for example, "I'm sure you don't really care about me. After all, you've never said that you did." The simple statement "I do care" would in this instance be less effective than a comment such as, "Might you not want to know that I care?" or, "Would it be hard for you to let yourself know how much I care?"

Cooling Things Down

At times of severe distress in the group, it may be necessary for the leaders to help the group move away from intense affect. This kind of modulation of affect may sometimes be necessary, for example, with more psychologically impaired patients—particularly in the early phases of group life when the safety of the group has not been adequately established.

Such "modulation techniques" include the following: (1) Periods of heated affect can be neutralized by introducing a more cognitive element. For example, the leader might ask patients about their thoughts (as opposed to their feelings), or might ask the group to make observations about what is currently going on in the group or what has transpired during the past few minutes. Similarly, leaders might summarize their own observations about what has transpired in the group. (2) Movement from a present focus to a past focus or from a past focus to a present focus can also be used to diffuse affect in the group. In much the same manner as the leader can move the group toward greater affect—choosing past or present focus in such a way as to elevate the feeling tone of the group—the leader can make the same choices in order to cool things down. For example, a patient involved in intense feelings about the past may be moved into a present focus by the leader asking whether she experiences any similar feelings toward current people in her life or toward people in the group (the choice, here, being to move toward the more neutral of the options). Similarly, the patient engaged in a present-focused heated exchange with another group member might be diverted, if it seems too intense for the group or for the particular member to handle, by asking her to think about what, from the past, this reaction might be hooking into.

These modulation techniques involve the leaders' selective use of distracting mechanisms (defensive maneuvers of sorts) to lower the intensity of affect. While these mechanisms are appropriate and useful on occasion (and, thus, are skills that leaders should know how to use), it is also important to recognize that, at times, the leaders' feelings that the group process needs to be neutralized may simply resonate with the group's feeling of being out of control. It is thus important for the leaders to be aware of their own countertransference reactions (discussed more fully in Chapter 10) before moving in too quickly to "cool things down."

Disengaging from the Struggle

At times the group leader may find that even his best attempts to maneuver the group out of an uncomfortable and unworkable impasse may not be effective. This may occur, for example, when two members seem to be mercilessly "going at one another" and the leaders' attempts to intercede are rebuffed, or when the group is engaged in a no-win battle with a particular patient who repeatedly breaks the group contract, dismissing the group's attempt to help get him back on track by becoming defensive but making no change in his behavior.

(This might occur, for example, with a patient who comes late each week with a "good excuse" and, when confronted, keeps insisting that he is well intentioned, to the group's continued rebuttals.) In such situations the leader may also find himself drawn into the struggle, feeling as if somehow he has to turn the situation around and fix the problem. Often, however, the pivotal point occurs when the therapist can disengage from the struggle, putting the responsibility back on the patient or the group. This is illustrated by the following example.

In a consultation that I did a few years ago with a couple who were considering joining my couples group, it became apparent after the first 15 minutes that neither husband nor wife had joined with me around any useful therapeutic purpose. They continued to carp at one another (pretty much keeping me out altogether) the entire time. All of my interventions were hostilely rebuffed or ignored, as the two continued their unrelenting criticism of one another. Finally, I gave up my repeated attempts to engage them and simply commented, "This doesn't seem to be going very well, does it? Perhaps we need to take a look at what's going on right here to decide whether it makes sense to proceed." At this, both patients rallied—indicating that they did want to try to work things out—and the session proceeded.

Although in a group session (unlike the couples consultation above) I would never suggest that the session might be ended because of an impasse, disengaging from a group struggle (and helping the group members take responsibility for turning things around) could be done in an analogous way. Thus, the leader might say, when two group members (or the group leader and a member) are engaged in a no-win battle, "This doesn't seem to be going very well, does it? Perhaps we need to take a look at what's going on to decide whether anything can be gained by continuing to proceed in this way."

This chapter has examined patient roadblocks that are expressed through deviations from the contract and through withholding defenses and disruptive defenses. Therapist techniques have also been discussed for dealing with each of these forms of resistance. The next chapter looks at resistance that emerges as the patient contemplates the final stage of group work and begins to consider termination.

❖ 9 ❖
Removing the Final Patient
Roadblock: Termination

Termination is the last phase of treatment, during which the patient will rework and put finishing touches on many of the issues he came for and will have an opportunity to learn how to say "good-bye"—an important recurring life task that is difficult for most people. For many patients (perhaps most), the prospect of terminating therapy is a complicated affair. Patients may raise the possibility of leaving before they are ready to go, may be ready to leave but uncertain about how to go about it, or may be fearful of the prospect of leaving and may regress when faced with the possibility of termination.

This chapter reviews the termination process, examining the ways in which patients bring it up, the possible meanings of termination for the patient, and strategies for therapeutically intervening both to help the patient make a constructive decision about whether or not he will leave and to help him through the actual termination process if he decides to leave.

Viewing the Termination Announcement as a Proposal to Be Considered

It is important to recognize that an announcement that somebody is terminating should be understood, not as a fait accompli, but as a communication that needs to be understood. When a patient comes in and says, "I've decided to leave in 3 weeks," some groups (and their leaders) transform this statement into a deed that has been accomplished. I find it more useful to understand such communications as a proposal that needs to be considered, and often the patient's way of raising other important issues. Thus, when I play back a patient's announcement, rather than phrasing it as "Your plan to leave in 3 weeks," I might be inclined to use softer language such as, "the possibility you have raised of leaving in 3 weeks," or "your proposed departure date." The idea is to keep the door open so the decision does not seem irreversible and more can be learned about what is going on.

It may be useful to remember that important relationships are often punctuated with thoughts about leaving or pronouncements of a plan to do so—sometimes in anger, sometimes when a relationship gets too hot. It is often, in fact, in the most important relationships that people need most to be able to reassure themselves that they can leave. But feeling able to leave is not the same thing as acting on it. Often, it is a way of communicating discomfort and serves as an indicator of something that needs to be addressed in the relationship.

Readiness for Termination

One way of exploring the issue which allows the therapist to collect more information about the patient's readiness or nonreadiness to leave, is for the therapist to ask the patient the following questions: (1) "What is it that you first came to work on?" and (2) "Where do things now stand with that?"

If the patient feels that there is still more to be done but that she "can't get at it any more," the therapist might ask, "What makes you feel there is still more to do? What are the indicators, in terms of the experiences that come up for you, that suggest that this is still a problem?" If the patient cannot produce much material, it may be that, indeed, at this point in the work the territory has been sufficiently covered. Sometimes, because of the therapist's own feelings about the termination or his own wishes for a more "perfect product," he may have difficulty accepting the idea of a termination.

When my patients begin to consider termination (particularly premature termination), I often find it useful to discuss with them the various ways that people leave a therapy group. I tell them that there are three points at which people generally think about leaving therapy, and that each is associated with different kinds of goal resolution, different feelings about leaving, and different ways of handling the termination. After reviewing these three routes of termination (gen-

erally in considerably fewer words than the descriptions I have outlined below), I ask the potential terminator to classify herself by indicating which of these categories she thinks her proposed termination
most closely matches. In most instances I find that patients are reasonably accurate in placing themselves or, at worst, put themselves between two categories (with one of the categories being the one I would
also see as the most likely). This provides a forum for discussing with
the patient where she is in her therapy.

The three categories of termination are as follows:

1. *Completers:* Completers have essentially finished the work
   that they came in for and are sufficiently educated regarding
   the benefits of group work that they understand, also, the
   impact of doing the last phase of work, saying good-bye. They
   also understand that saying good-bye is a process—something
   that we all need to learn how to do better—and that the
   therapy group offers a unique opportunity to learn how to do
   this. These patients are able to review their goals and gains in
   therapy as well as reflect upon their losses, as they think about
   giving up the group and how it will feel, ultimately, to be gone.
2. *Plateauers:* These patients have done some of the work that
   they came in for but have a sense that they are not really
   finished. Rather, for the time being, they are "stuck." Plateauers have no clear sense of what more can be accomplished at
   the present time. (Often these patients return to treatment at
   a later point.) These patients are able to do some of the work
   of saying good-bye, although usually in a more abbreviated
   way than completers. The good-byes serve as the last focused
   project that the patient can gain from working on.
3. *Fleers:* (This group may also be referred to as "Flyers") These
   patients experience a pressing need to "get out." In fact, the
   pressure to leave is often the telling signal of the fleer. Such
   patients cannot take the time to terminate, but rather, feel
   tremendous pressure to leave in haste. Generally patients in
   this category are avoiding something in the group, or in themselves, that they feel uncomfortable about and from which they
   wish to flee as rapidly as possible.

The patient who is considering a rapid exit from the group may be
encouraged to stay longer—at least long enough to consider whether,

in fact, she is making the right decision—by commenting "One of the characteristics of a good decision is that it remains a good decision even after consideration a few weeks later." Generally, I take the position that the patient's proposed departure may make sense at this point, but that until we explore it we will not fully understand why she is choosing to leave now, or whether, in fact, this is the right time.

Another route for dealing with a patient who is facing the possibility of termination is to inquire what the patient believes she might work on if she remained in the group. Sometimes this is a way of getting at what the patient might be avoiding or taking flight from. Sometimes it may simply confirm that the patient does not feel in sufficient pain at the moment to warrant further continuation in therapy or that perhaps the work is, in fact, essentially done.

The Termination Process

Termination is the last phase of the therapeutic work. The patient who takes time to leave appropriately has an opportunity to put the finishing touches on the work that he came to do originally and has an opportunity to learn to effectively say "good-bye". Some of the important aspects of the termination process are the following:

1. The departing member will be able to solicit and hear feedback from other group members about how they feel about his leaving, including possible views about why he may need to stay a bit longer.
2. The departing member will review what he came to work on in the group and how well he has done with each of his goals. In the process, he will reminisce about the group, recalling the past and noting changes that he recalls in others in the group, as well as himself.
3. Alongside of charting the progress that he has made, the departing member will explore disappointed hopes about the things that have not changed.
4. The entire group will have an opportunity to page through the scrapbook of time, fondly remembering—an important part of the termination process.
5. The departing member will have an opportunity to say something to each member of the group, connecting to each, as he

says good-bye—what they have meant to him, his hopes for their future, etc. (and group members will have an opportunity to share the same with the departing member).

6. The departing member, in the process of saying good-bye, will have an opportunity to rework and touch up the original issues that brought him into treatment. It is helpful to let patients know that it is common in the termination phase for the original issues and conflicts to be reexperienced. The termination phase presents an opportunity to face the conflicts once again, to put the finishing touches on understanding what they are about, and to metabolize this understanding.

7. Finally, the departing member should be encouraged to think about those things he fears will not be said before he leaves (both the things that he fears others in the group will not be able to say to him and the things that he feels that he might not be able to say to them). Of course, in the process of talking about this, most of these things will be said.

Sometimes I help patients with this last step by asking, the last session or so before their departure, "What do you imagine, as you're walking down the hill following your last session, that you may regret not having said to the group or to a particular member?" Or, "What do you imagine wishing that you might have heard that never got said?" One of the most common responses to this is for the patient to express concerns about not knowing whether the group leader cared (since she has "never said that she did"). When this comes up, I might inquire, "Are there other ways that you might know that I care?" Or, "How could you not know that I care?"

My stance in such circumstances is to continue processing with the patient—often embedding in the stem of my question the affirmative statement that he wants to hear. (For example, in the previous questions the stem of the sentence says that I do care.) I believe that these messages are heard in a more lasting and meaningful way than a simple assertion such as, "Of course I do care," or, "Yes, I will miss you." The latter statements are often too close to familiar social dialogue—words that are often said lightly and are easily dismissed. Instead, the question, "How could you not know that I care?" or, "What makes it so hard to take in that I care?" leaves the patient in a processing mode—considering and reflecting upon his feelings rather than simply dealing with the assertion of the therapist. The dialogue can be continued.

Termination and Feelings of Abandonment

For some patients, termination may feel like an abandonment. Even the patient who enters a short-term group in which he knows in advance that his stay will be limited to 6 months may feel as if he is being abandoned by the therapist and the group when it comes time for him to terminate. Similarly, the patient who raises the issue of termination himself after a prolonged therapeutic relationship (individual or group) may feel abandoned if his thoughts about termination are too readily accepted. The issue of termination may be raised as a "test" to see if people care enough to persuade the group member to stay. This is illustrated by the following case example:

After several years of couples therapy, Mrs. X began to talk about all the areas in which she and her husband had made headway and to suggest that they should probably be thinking about terminating. Since the timing of her suggestion seemed appropriate (she and her husband had been doing much better for several months), as did their discussions about termination, I empathically failed Mrs. X by not recognizing her need (unstated) to have me hang on to her and her husband a bit longer. It was not until the day that we terminated, when she handed me a gift and an extremely sweet (reaction-formed) thank you note, that I realized that she was enraged at me. As we talked about the message communicated through the gift, it became clear that Mrs. X (who had lost both of her parents during the course of our 4 years together) had felt that since things between her and her husband were better, it would be "babyish" to continue in therapy. However, alongside of this was also a powerful wish to keep me. Her hope had been that I would tell them that they were not ready to go. When I failed to do this, she felt terribly abandoned by me and experienced it as if I were actually kicking them out.

When I asked the couple more about the thoughts and feelings that might be communicated by the gift, their initial response proclaimed their great appreciation for all I had done. To my further inquiries, "In addition to the feelings of appreciation that you have, I wonder if there might be some other feelings that you might have about me and about your leaving," Mrs. X responded, "Well, I guess you wanted us to leave and thought we were ready." To this I responded, "Perhaps you have

*been feeling that I encouraged you to leave a little before you were ready,
and that I should have resisted a bit more when you suggested the idea."
The patient quietly nodded in the affirmative. Although I suggested a few
more sessions to explore this a bit more and to reach a more comfortable
closure, the couple declined, having filled our hour with an Adult Education class that they had signed up for together.*

The Patient's Reluctance to Grow (and Go)

For some patients termination is highly conflictual since it implies
getting better and leaving behind many things that are familiar, even
if not totally adaptive. Getting better means change and does not
always feel unambiguously positive. After all, the prospect of being big
and grown is a mixed blessing. The nurturance and support—the kind
of caring that was present when one felt vulnerable, helpless, and
child-like—suddenly may feel as if it will vanish as one achieves desired "adulthood" (just as when we reach a certain age, there is an
expectation that we leave home and move on, getting on without the
old supports that we have been used to). Even for patients whose life
styles have been maladaptive in many ways and whose relationships
have been complicated, growing up and leaving behind one's old ways
may be associated with loosing the only supports they have known.

For some patients this may result in feeling stuck as they near
termination and the last phase of work that they need to do in the
group. The very act of labeling "the last phase" may be frightening,
since the prospect of accomplishing this final task is connected to
having to leave the group. Thus, stuckness, possibly even regression,
may occur as the patient defines himself as "nearing the end." It is thus
important that the group leader be sensitive to this potential dynamic
and open to exploring it, particularly when patients seem regressed or
reluctant to move.

Knowing That One Can Leave: A Ticket to Feeling Safe
about Sharing

Many patients raise the issue of leaving to assure themselves that it is
possible for them to exit, and may share important and intimate
material only after announcing impending departure. For such pa-

tients, knowing that the door remains open makes it safe to stay and open up.

> *Mr. G, a year after joining his long-term group, was still finding it hard to really open up. He felt there was, as he put it, "stuff stuck in my craw that I want to get out." After lamenting this condition for some weeks, he spontaneously went off for a 1-week therapy group—a time-limited retreat away from home—and came back to his long-term group impressed with how much he had shared and how wonderful the short-term group had been. For this man, a time-limited experience that he knew would soon come to an end offered the perfect opportunity to feel safe enough to open up. He returned to his long-term therapy group, disappointed that he had not been able to share with them and feeling that now he had good reason to finally leave (since in comparison with the 1-week institute, the group paled miserably). The leader appropriately interpreted Mr. G's concerns about the safety of getting close when there was no readily perceived exit, a theme that had relevance for the entire group, as one member after another worried about whether they would finally be able to leave the group and wanted reassurance that they could exit if they needed to.*

Premature Termination

The Goldilocks Theory

People leave therapy prematurely when there is either "too much" or "too little." When what is going on is essentially "just right," the patient stays (until she is ready to terminate). The "too little" or "too much" may have to do with feelings of connection (not enough, or more than the patient can handle), changes that are being made (too little, or more than what one is ready for), or other dimensions that are relevant for a given patient. Another way of understanding this is to think about the fact that when people first raise the issue of termination, this may occur because they are not feeling sufficiently connected. Conversely, it may occur because they are feeling too connected and are aware that at some point they will have to leave and fear becoming overly dependent. Rather than experiencing the dependency feelings and weathering them, they decide that now is as good a time as any to leave. Thus, it is often helpful to ask the patient who is prematurely considering termination whether it is because she feels that she is not connected enough or whether, perhaps, she feels too connected?

Helping the Patient to Articulate Disappointment

Often, the patient who proposes to leave the group prematurely is making a statement about his disappointment in the group. In particular, the patient who is quiet and seemingly never quite engaged with the group may be expressing his disappointed yearnings—yearnings for the kind of attachment and engagement that he sees among others in the group but which have never materialized for him.

An example of this kind of disappointed relationship with the group recently came to my attention. A middle-aged man had been in his group for about 11 months—always somewhat on the periphery and minimally engaged. Several weeks after being confronted by the group about his peripheral position, he came back to the group announcing that he had decided to leave since "I still did not know why I drank and I think that another group might be more helpful." Although the group had, on many occasions, articulated their disappointment with him (along with an invitation for him to participate in a different way), until this member raised the possibility of terminating, he had not even hinted at his own disappointment.

With such a patient it might be helpful to explore the patient's disappointment. The leader may say, "It sounds like you've been kind of disappointed in this group—that there were things that you were hoping for that you still haven't gotten." The leader might then ask, "Can you say more about how you think things might go differently for you in another group?" Helping this patient to articulate his disappointment with the group (how he wished things had been different) may also provide a useful forum for other group members, who may themselves feel somewhat disappointed in the group. To this patient I might say, "I think it might be real helpful for you, as well as others in here, to talk about some of the ways that you feel that the group, or I, have let you down. Because my hunch is that others in here have also felt disappointed from time to time and are aware that there are things they wish they were getting that don't seem to come about in here."

It might also be useful to note that an important part of the work of termination, even when it is not premature, is for the departing member to have a chance to explore disappointed hopes—fantasies about things that might have changed but still haven't—alongside of the progress and gains that have been made. In any case, it is important that the group leader be prepared to listen for disappointment, especially when the issue of termination is raised.

Premature Termination Related to Breaks in the Contract

The patient who decides to depart in a manner that runs counter to her contract with the group (e.g., allowing less than the 3 weeks stated in the ground rules) can often benefit by an opportunity to examine issues around commitment. For such a patient it may be possible to reframe the issue around her style of departure so that it fits with major life issues that she can profitably explore in the group. The therapist might indicate to such a patient that although leaving the group may still be an appropriate decision, if she takes enough time to process it appropriately—the next 3 weeks, as initially agreed—she will be in a better position to make this decision and will also understand more about the way that she handles commitments. The leader might say, "It might be helpful for you to think about the fact that you made a contract with the group about how you were going to terminate, and I'm wondering how it feels to be giving up on something you have committed yourself to. Clearly this is not the only situation in which this comes up for you. For example, you have let us know that you have frequently have a hard time getting places on time or completing projects at work. If you come back another few times, we might have an opportunity to explore the ways that you let yourself and others down after you have made a commitment."

The Patient Who Raises Termination When Her Insurance Money Is Up

Occasionally a patient raises the issue of leaving group when her insurance money is up—suggesting that whatever it was that she was getting was fine "as long as it didn't cost anything." When this comes up, I am inclined to challenge the notion that it has not yet cost anything—since there are always considerable expenditures, aside from money, associated with being in therapy. Thus, I might say to such a patient, "Actually, you have already made a considerable investment in your treatment—setting other things aside to be here and making this a priority in your life, even though at times it took a tremendous amount of effort to get here, given the problems you were having with your car, the long commute, child care conflicts, etc. What was your hope when you began making this investment about what you would get from the group?" I would then attempt to help the patient remember the goals that she had set for herself in the pregroup interview and to review her progress with these goals in relation to her wish to exit at this point. It is important to remember that moves to terminate, especially hastily, often occur at the cutting edge of treatment. The thought of leaving often comes up just as a patient is about to encounter a major conflict area (often the very one that she has come to work on); and if the patient can be engaged at these points, there is an opportunity for real growth and progress. The following case example illustrates this kind of no-money termination proposal at the cutting edge of treatment.

Mrs. B, in her pregroup interview, stated that she wanted to work on issues around intimacy. When the therapist asked her to define more specifically how this currently was a problem for her, she stated, "Well, my husband and I married when I was 18—because that was pretty much expected in our neighborhood. But as the years have gone on, I realize that I don't love him and that we are basically "two strangers passing in the night"—but, oddly enough, this is not a problem for me." Mrs. B was thus expressing her conflict about intimacy—on the one hand thinking that perhaps she would like to get closer, but on the other, feeling that the current distance between her and her husband was OK. In the group, at the point she raised the possibility of leaving ("because of money"), she had been getting increasingly close to other members and had begun to share a considerable amount of emotionally charged personal material. Most recently she had shared that she had decided to act on her feelings of estrangement from her husband by moving to a third-floor bedroom. But this lasted for only one night, as she realized that she couldn't sleep without him." Conflicted about her wishes for intimacy and fears of dependency, she explained to the group that she had returned downstairs, "recognizing that I needed him physically." As in her pregroup interview, when she talked about lack of intimacy and then stated, "this is no problem" (implying conflict about getting closer), we see her moving up to the attic to take distance yet returning to her husband's room—more dependent on him than she was prepared to acknowledge. The group leader pointed out that this member had, particularly recently, been sharing a great deal in the group and seemed to be getting a good deal out of it, and that her suggestion of termination might be seen as a *sort of "move to the attic" in the group. That is, that she was somehow aware that the group meant something to her (just as she was with her marriage) and aware of some feelings of attachment, but felt conflicted about those attachments.*

The Patient Who Wants to Leave Group in Order to Demonstrate Her Autonomy

Sometimes premature termination is posed by a patient as an indicator of her ability to "stand on her own two feet" and "make her own decisions." This patient has taken what seems like a single autonomous step by expressing the wish to leave and her willingness to do this, even if others do not agree. This step, in a sense, is a signal of the issue that she needs to work on but is clearly not an adequate, integrated solution. However, her raising the issue in this way suggests that there may be a part of her that wants to begin to address it. The initial group task is to get her to delay her departure long enough to see whether the group may be able to help her with this piece of work—at least staying long enough to understand more about what the departure is all about. I might say to this patient, "You are letting us know that there is something important here for us to work on—the wish to feel that you are a person who can make your own decisions and will not be dominated by others. I suspect that your raising this issue expresses, in part, a wish to deal with it, but you won't have that opportunity if you leave now."

When issues of autonomy and independence get merged with termination issues, the patient often finds herself in a bind in which an unnegotiated departure is experienced as the only way to make the point, "I can do what I want; I don't have to be influenced by others." This creates a situation in which the only way that she can feel that she is doing what she wants, ironically, is by doing something else that she may not want to do. The work, then, involves helping the patient to figure out whether she can do what she wants and also stay in the group. Sometimes reframing the conflict is helpful, suggesting, "It sounds like it is important for you to know that you can leave and that the situation that you are setting up with us now is a way of helping to clarify that you can decide to do what you want. Once you have settled that, perhaps you will not need to actually leave."

Part and parcel of this autonomy struggle is a message that is usually communicated to other group members that any feedback which they provide will be either ignored or repudiated, since to do otherwise would prove that the patient is not adequately autonomous but still "people-pleasing as always." To such a patient I might say, "It probably would not be a good idea to stay just because other people want you to; but what if you come to think that it would be a good idea to stay?" This helps the individual to save face. She can decide, "I am staying because I want to." Or, I might say, "If you decided yourself that it might be useful, do you think that you could stay a while longer—at least long enough to understand some of the complicated things that are going on for you right now?" Or, I might ask, "If you started having second thoughts about all this and decided that it might make sense to stay a little longer, would you be able to change your mind?" If a group member says, "No," her response clearly would be an indication of "digging in one's heels" rather than demonstrating health and readiness to leave. If, on the other hand, she felt that she might be able to change her mind if she felt that it made sense, I might ask, "What kind of information or input do you think might be useful in helping you to think about this in a different way?" This is an important question because this individual has already set up the situation in such a way that she will reject most feedback from the group for fear of "people pleasing."

For some patients the autonomy issue is especially likely to surface at times in which the patient is feeling particularly dependent on the group and fearful that if he does not leave now, he will never have an opportunity—"that I will be here forever." For such patients I might say, "It sounds like it is important for you to reassure yourself that you could leave, but I wonder if leaving is the only way that you can assure yourself of that?" Or I might say, "Of course you can leave—but do you need to exercise that option in order to know that you can do it?"

As the examples above illustrate, at turning points in treatment patients often bring up pivotal issues from which, if they stay, they have an opportunity to grow. However, if they flee, they have merely signaled the issue without having addressed it. Suggestions to terminate are often the harbinger of these turning points, and if we understand the conflict that is being represented, we have a particularly good opportunity to help the patient move to another level of work. The group member who prematurely raises termination gives the group an opportunity either to help him grow or to lose him as a member. Thus, the therapy will proceed with a flourish, or the patient will flee from, or plateau himself out of, therapy.

Sometimes at such turning points, patients themselves may have a sense that something further could be done—but feel that they would like to leave for now with the option of returning. I would initially address this by stating, "It sounds as if you have your own doubts about whether leaving makes sense right now, or about whether you have completed the work. I think it's important that we have an opportunity to think more about the doubts and the mixed feelings."

When a patient who has decided to leave asks about the possibility of returning in the future, I would respond, "The decision about whether or not you might be able to rejoin this group depends, to a large extent, on the way in which you leave. This means that you give yourself and the group enough time to talk about your departure so that we have some understanding about what's motivating you to leave at this point and how future work might go were you to return." I am thus letting the patient know that he can not simply beat a hasty retreat now and expect later on to come back no matter what. (This would be particularly important to stress for a patient who is giving the group insufficient notice.) I would also let him know that returning to the group would depend on whether there was an opening in the group at the point he wished to return, what the group was working on, and how well his issues and situation fit in with what was going on in the group.

The Dwindling Patient

The patient who seems to be dealing with termination by gradually dwindling away needs to be attended to early on. Such patients may come one week and cancel the next few sessions, come again for a session followed by one or two uncanceled absences. Sometimes patients who are ready to terminate may test whether it feels OK to leave by such punctuated attendance. Others may begin to punctuate their attendance when issues become heated in the group and group participation begins to feel frightening. For still others, such punctuated attendance may reflect disappointment in the group and ambivalence about continuing, which if not addressed by the group may lead to premature departure. Regardless of the dynamics involved in the punctuated attendance, the patient who dwindles away should not be ignored. Outreach phone calls and, ultimately, a letter, if phone calls are not responded to, may be important in helping the patient feel that his absence has been noted. Such outreach may not only make a great deal of difference in recruiting this individual back into the group but, in addition, is important to the group as a whole in terms of clearly reaffirming the group boundaries (people who are in the group must come) and letting the group know that the leaders take seriously patients' commitment to the group. It is also important to remember that the manner in which we deal with the patient's absences (and ultimate departure if that is what follows) may influence his willingness to reengage in treatment in the future.

This chapter has examined the resistances in the patient that emerge as termination from the group is contemplated, as well as resistances that are reflected in premature departures. The next chapter looks at roadblocks in the therapist that complicate the group's journey.

❖ *10* ❖
Removing the Roadblocks in the Therapist

The therapist who is well prepared and well trained will be most able to effectively guide his group on its journey. The well-prepared leader will understand his own issues and how these interact with the issues of group members and will be ready to examine myths and misconceptions that he holds that may interfere with the group's maximizing its potential. The group's effectiveness is diminished not only by limitations in the leader's skill (hence the need for training, discussed in the next chapter) but also by anything that impairs the leader's ability to listen sensitively and respond to the clinical material. In this chapter such roadblocks in the leader are discussed in terms of: (1) therapist's countertransference reactions (and ways that they resonate with personal issues in the life of the therapist); (2) confusion about the therapeutic stance—how active to be, when, and around what issues; and (3) common snafus that leaders frequently encounter. In addition, issues related to co-leadership are addressed, including some of the pros and cons, selection of a co-leader, and care and maintenance of the co-therapy relationship.

COUNTERTRANSFERENCE ISSUES

The group leader's countertransference reactions, if understood, can be a tremendous asset in furthering the work of the therapy. If not understood or recognized, these feelings can serve as serious roadblocks for the therapist. In the material that follows, countertransference is defined, signs of countertransference are provided, and examples are given of the ways in which countertransference reactions are negatively reflected in breaks in the therapeutic contract, or can be positively and productively utilized by making use of projective identification.

Countertransference Defined

Countertransference, in its broadest terms, may be conceptualized as "the total emotional reaction of the therapist to the patient, with consideration of the (therapist's) entire range of conscious, preconscious, and unconscious attitudes, beliefs, and feelings . . ." (Imhof, Hirsch, & Terenzi, 1983, p. 492). As this definition suggests, countertransference is a fact of life for the therapist. When properly understood, it can guide and inform our therapeutic work and can serve as one of the most important tools we have in understanding what is going on for the patient. If not understood or recognized, these feelings often get in the way of successful therapeutic work.

There are several ways of looking at the different aspects of countertransference and at the roots of the various feelings that our patients stir up in us. Winnicott's (1949) distinction is one of the most useful. He differentiates between "objective" and "subjective" countertransference reactions.

Subjective Countertransference: "Subjective" reactions are the reactions that the patient creates in the therapist that relate to the therapist's own past and his own personal idiosyncrasies. (We might also think of these subjective reactions as a sort of "transference" that the therapist has to the patient or to the group.) These countertransference feelings, if not adequately attended to, get in the way of the therapeutic work. Subjective countertransference, though hopefully minimized both through the therapist's own personal psychotherapy and through supervision, remains an inevitable part of clinical work. For this reason, self-reflection and continuous self-monitoring are necessary. The more we know about our wishes, attitudes, inclinations, and prejudices, the more likely we are to understand what is going on and to be able to use our understanding in a way that is helpful to our patients.

Objective Countertransference: "Objective" countertransference reactions, on the other hand, refer to feelings that the patient induces in the therapist that are relevant to the patient's core conflicts and issues. Understanding these induced feelings can pave the way to learning about aspects of the patient's inner life and ways of relating to others that might otherwise be hard to appreciate. As Levine (1988) points out, by creating this differentiation between subjective and objective countertransference, Winnicott directed therapists' attention to the interaction between patient and therapist as a productive arena for exploring important aspects of the patient's dynamics.

Objective countertransference can be divided into two major categories. The first category consists of therapist's feelings that are in reaction to the transference feelings of the patient. Here the patient treats the therapist as if she were some other significant actor in his life. Or put another way, he projects onto the therapist feelings that belong to a significant other from the past. An example might be the patient reacting to the therapist angrily, as if she were the bad withholding mother of his past—leading the therapist to feel that she is being viewed unfairly and that whatever she does will be seen as inadequate. The therapist's reactions to her own feelings may then include thoughts of modifying her clinical approach so as not to be viewed in such a negative light. As Searles (1979) points out,

> . . . when the analyst is being unaccustomedly warmly participative with the patient, we have a clue to the analyst's unconsciously avoiding the negative transference role in which the patient is tending to perceive him (as being, say, a perceivably remote and unfeeling parent). (p. 579)

The second category consists of therapist's feelings that are set into motion by the therapist's ability to resonate with important feelings that the patient experiences about himself. This category includes: (1) feelings of the patient that the therapist directly identifies with, and which by attention to her own emotional response, will help her identify with what the patient is feeling (for example, the therapist is feeling very sad and understands this to be what the patient is feeling); and (2) feelings that arise in the therapist when the patient projects unwanted aspects of himself onto the therapist, who then takes them in and experiences them as her own. Racker (1968) clarified the distinction between these two differential countertransference responses to the patient's feelings about himself, labeling them *concordant* and *complementary identifications, respectively.*

Concordant identifications are more readily perceived, leading to a direct empathic response (except in those instances in which the therapist herself is defending against knowing the patient's painful feelings). The therapist directly experiences the same feeling as the patient—the patient is sad, the therapist feels the sadness; the patient is enraged at his mother who has abused him terribly, and the therapist experiences that rage, as well.

Complementary identifications occur through a somewhat more complicated process. To understand this, Racker makes use of the concept of projective identification, a process whereby the patient expels and ejects aspects of himself into the therapist. Although the concept of projective identification has been elaborated in a number of different ways in the literature, Levine's (1988) concise summary of Malin and Grotstein's (1966) conceptualization highlights the importance of investigating the interaction between the patient and therapist. Thus, according to Levine, in projective identification,

> there is an unconscious fantasy of projecting a part of oneself into another person . . .; [and] there is a pressure exerted through the interpersonal interaction such that the recipient of the projection experiences pressure to think, feel, and behave congruently with the projection. (p. 99)

Thus, in projective identification, the therapist is induced by the patient to experience many of the unacceptable feelings that the patient experiences about himself. That is, the patient projects out unacceptable aspects of himself in a way such that the therapist identifies with them and experiences them as her own—feeling, and perhaps even acting, as if the projection were accurate. As Grotstein (1981) puts it,

> Powerful feelings are more often than not expressed by giving another person the experience of how one feels. . . . All human beings seem to have the need . . . to be relieved of the burden of unknown, unknowable feelings by being able to express them, literally as well as figuratively into the flesh, so to speak, of the other so that this other person can know how one felt. . . . We each are projectors and ultimately wish the other to know the experience (that) we cannot communicate . . . until we have been convinced that the other understands. We cannot be convinced that they understand until we are convinced that they now contain the experience. (pp. 202–203)

This kind of reaction, if understood and appropriately responded to by the therapist, can be extremely useful in helping the patient, not only to feel understood, but also to come to tolerate and accept these feelings within himself. The therapist gets into trouble when she fails to understand that her own feelings and reactions provide important data about the patient. This is especially likely if the therapist herself has unexplored conflicts in similar areas and can no longer keep track of what is hers and what is the patient's.

As an example of projective identification we might consider a therapist's reaction to a patient who insists that he is "getting worse" and that the therapist is "useless" and perhaps even "damaging." The therapist, in reaction to the patient's onslaught, responds with anxiety, comes to feel helpless, inadequate, and incompetent, and perhaps even comes to view herself as dangerous or harmful. It is at this point that the therapist has come to understand and to experience how the patient views himself. The patient feels incompetent and inadequate, and he projects these unacceptable aspects of himself onto the therapist by accusing her of "not understanding him," "failing to make him better," and perhaps "making him even worse." The therapist, resonating with these feelings that are being projected onto her, in turn begins to feel incompetent with this particular patient, to wonder if she knows what she is doing, and to worry that perhaps she is making the patient worse. Some of her fears may even be enacted as she, in fact, begins to actually make mistakes—to fluster and to blunder in ways that are otherwise not characteristic. This validates the patient's projections and completes the interactive loop.

What can also be seen from this brief example is that projective identification, in contrast to simple projection, involves two people and is truly dyadic in nature. As Levine (1988) points out, projective identification is distinguished from projection "in its reliance on the other person's active participation in the defensive operation" (p. 99). Projection need only involve a single person—the projector. It can operate in a vacuum. Unacceptable feelings can be projected out, even onto inanimate objects (such as magazine pictures). No reciprocal reaction is required. Thus, for example, an angry, hostile patient may see others (including the therapist) as angry and hostile in the absence of any particular confirming behavior on the part of these others. In contrast, projective identification occurs in an interactional context. There is a dyadic interaction in which the patient puts out unacceptable aspects of himself (the projection), and the therapist receives this (and in some way identifies or resonates with it) and acts or feels accordingly. Two people are involved; and the therapist, by understanding what is going on between herself and the patient, has a unique opportunity to understand important aspects of the patient's dynamics.

An example of projective identification that captures something of the subtlety and complexity of the process is provided in Searles' (1979) description of the intense reactions to a particular patient, "a highly intelligent, intensely ambitious lawyer."

> I found myself immersed in deeply troubled feelings concerning my sense of identity as an analyst. I had a nagging feeling, from the beginning of our work, that I was unable to keep up with the rapid and abundant flow of analytic material from him. He typically reported dreams which were not only numerous but which clearly possessed much significance for the analysis, and he himself was able to perceive their significances more rapidly than I could. I felt that this man. . . was only highlighting a chronic and pervasive deficiency of mine as an analyst. . . .
>
> It came to me as an immense relief . . . to discover that an important cause of my troubled feelings consisted in his transference to me as being his own small-child self, the youngest child among several siblings, a child who had felt chronically unable to keep up not only with his highly competitive older and larger siblings, but also with his mother. . . . (p. 579)

Importance of a Continuously Self-Reflective Stance

From all that we have pointed to in the discussions above, it is clear that the therapist who works most effectively with his patients will be one who can maintain a continuously self-reflective stance, examining his own feelings and attitudes in response to the patient. In the interaction between the patient and therapist, it is essential to continuously monitor the dynamic process and interaction between the two—what the patient projects out, what belongs to the therapist, and the interaction between the two. As Imhof et al. (1983) suggest, one's own personal therapy experience is an invaluable aid in this task, as is supervision.

> Given the endemic and epidemic nature of substance abuse in society today, it is no longer unlikely that a member of the therapist's family may have a serious problem with drug abuse, including alcoholism. In such instances, there is an even greater need for height-

ened awareness of countertransferential and attitudinal derivatives emanating from the therapist's personal life. It is imperative to recognize to what extent, if any, a therapist's own personal issues become intertwined with the separate treatment issues of the patient, and in this area clinical supervision can again play a most significant role. (pp. 507–508)

Cutting across the various kinds of countertransference, it should be noted that regardless of whether we are talking about objective or subjective countertransference, at times the therapist will initially be more aware of the defense *against* his countertransference feelings than of the countertransference feelings themselves. For example, the therapist may be aware of feeling excessively conciliatory as a defense against his countertransference rage, or the therapist may be aware of feeling overly concerned about "helping and caretaking" in the face of an angry, denigrating patient who is accusing the therapist of being "worthless." In these instances it takes careful self-reflection and self-scrutiny to understand the countertransference feeling and its meaning for the patient.

It should also be noted that the distinctions between subjective and objective countertransference, as well as any of the other countertransference distinctions that we have made, are independent of whether countertransference reactions get in the way or not. Any countertransference reaction that is not understood impedes the work of the therapy—subjective, because it may actually obscure or get in the way of understanding the patient; objective, because valuable information about the patient and her interactions are lost.

Heightened Countertransference Reactions in Group Psychotherapy

It should be clear from the discussion above that when we are talking about countertransference feelings, we are not talking about "good" or "bad" reactions on the part of the therapist. Rather, we are talking about the therapist's reactions to and resonation with the patient, and the importance of understanding these reactions in order to maximize therapeutic effectiveness. Although the potential for powerful reactions to the patient and resonance with her material also exists in individual therapy, this kind of resonance is often particularly intense in group therapy. I liken this to the infinitely greater number of possibilities for resonance that occur in a large chamber ensemble compared to a single instrument playing the same tune. The more parts or voices, the greater the potential for resonance.

Signals of Countertransference

Tip-offs to the presence of countertransference can be found by monitoring both the covert and overt responses of the therapist. Covert responses include changes in the therapist's thoughts or feelings: (1) unexpected shifts in attitude toward the patient that feel somewhat capricious to the therapist; (2) preoccupation with a given patient or group as expressed through dreams, recurring thoughts, or rehashes in one's head about a session or a portion of a session (i.e., the feeling that one cannot get a particular patient, or group, out of one's mind); and (3) feeling mired down, exhausted, or stuck or having fantasies about missing a session. Overt responses are reflected in the therapist's actions: (1) stereotyped or fixed responses to the patient despite variations in the material that the patient brings in or how he presents it; (2) inappropriate affective responses to the patient (i.e., responses that differ from the therapist's usual behavior); and (3) changes in the therapeutic contract—therapist lateness, sleepiness during the hour, changing the time of appointments or cutting them short, neglecting to return phone calls, and laxness about the patient's failure to respect the therapeutic contract.

As Langs (1975) indicates, the manner in which the basic framework and and boundaries of the therapeutic setting are managed (or mismanaged) provides important information about the countertransferential reactions of the therapist. That is, whenever the basic therapeutic contract is broken or the ground rules are modified by either the patient or the therapist, the specter of countertransference is raised. Obviously, examining these kinds of modifications will be facilitated if the therapist and the patient have a clear idea of what the basic ground rules are. Appendix F provides a detailed checklist taken from Vannicelli (1989) that summarizes important dimensions of the therapeutic contract in terms of what is expected of the patient and what is expected of the therapist. These expectations or ground rules become a screen against which the therapist can measure deviations in therapeutic procedure.

Unfortunately, confusion about the ground rules is not uncommon among therapists and contributes to even greater confusion and frustration when the patient appears to be breaking one (or is he?). It is thus a good idea, when first beginning with a patient, to have a checklist that covers aspects of the contract that you want to be sure that you cover with the patient and about which you have made systematic notations to yourself. Often, the face sheet that you use for documenting the patient's name, address, and phone numbers as well as insurance information and party to contact in case of emergency can also provide an area for noting aspects of the working agreement that you have made explicit with the patient (such as fee, policy regarding payment for missed sessions, length of the hour, when fee increases will be negotiated, how payment will be handled). This information should be placed at the beginning of each patient's chart (see Appendix G for a sample face sheet) so that at any point at which a deviation or infraction seems to have occurred, you can check your face sheet to see whether it is a part of the agreement that has already been articulated. You may also want to note on this document whether a copy of the group ground rules were handed out to the patient and whether or not they were reviewed in detail in the pregroup interview.

Changing the Ground Rules

Although it is important to have a clear set of ground rules so that both the patient and therapist know what to expect, there will be times when it may be appropriate for the therapist to modify her behavior. For example, when a patient is in crisis, it may be indicated to see him more often or to extend the session. However, even an "obvious" change such as this should be thought about carefully. As Langs (1975) cautions in his detailed discussion about the importance of maintaining a consistent clinical framework,

> . . . deviations . . . should be limited to . . . relatively rare clinical situations . . . (after) the therapist's countertransference has been carefully subjected to self-analysis . . . . Before deviating, a full consideration of all other disturbing factors should be made, since problems within the therapist and with his technique are often more important to the stalemate than the psychopathology of the patient.
> In . . . those circumstances where the therapist formulates the need for a deviation . . . he should counterbalance his assessment of

the indications for the deviation with a full anticipation of the possible negative consequences. (pp. 118–119)

Often, when the therapist is tempted to break from his usual policy—for example, extending or increasing the sessions or changing the therapy hour in some other way—his impulse to do something different is directly related to things that are going on in the therapeutic interaction. Although, undoubtedly, there will be times that it will be appropriate for the therapist to follow his instincts and modify his procedure in some way, it is often wise, before acting impulsively, to take a few days to think about it.

When Leaders Must Break a Rule

Although clear ground rules for the conduct and maintenance of the group are essential, occasional deviations from the ground rules—introduced either by the group leaders or by the members—are inevitable. It is important, whenever a deviation occurs, that it is used as an opportunity to simultaneously reassert the importance of the ground rule and the way in which the particular deviation is an exception. If this is not done, the deviation itself becomes part of the new norms of the group and the original ground rule loses some of its effectiveness. Thus, if because of some crisis or urgent issue in the group, the leaders feel that it is important to extend the group time by a few minutes, this should be done by first reestablishing that the boundary is important, and then by indicating that there is something else going on that makes it essential to modify that boundary in this particularly instance. If possible, it is also helpful to set a new boundary for the deviation, as well. For example:

> In one of our groups, as the time neared for the session to end, it became apparent that two members had been drinking. The leaders, concerned that specific contracts be renegotiated with both patients (along with precise plans for new supports that would be embraced during the week), felt that it would be important to finish this business before the group members departed. Thus, one leader said to the other, "I'm concerned that we only have a few minutes left tonight, but also feel that it's important that we have a chance to reach closure on some of the important issues that have come up. Although I think it's very important

that we begin and end on time, I wonder how the group would feel about remaining an extra 10 minutes so that we can rework the contracts for the two members who have had drinking slips. " Thus, there was not simply a deviation that went unnoted, or a casual slippage of a rule, but a rather deliberate attempt to deal with a current crisis by renegotiating a new ending time for that one evening. The renegotiation also has the advantage of letting group members know how much longer the group would be extended, thus providing a new clear boundary.

When Patients' Slip-Ups Parallel Similar Slip-Ups by the Therapist

Therapists often find it particularly difficult to bring up boundary infractions in the group that parallel infractions that they, themselves, have made. For example, it is common to hear in supervision, "I walked into the group 3 minutes late, and two or three patients trickled in after I did. I thought I should have dealt with their lateness, but how could I, after being late myself?" Clearly, this is an understandable sentiment on the part of the therapist. It feels uncomfortable to call someone else on a faux pas that we ourselves have committed. On the other hand, therapists are human. We occasionally make mistakes, we accidentally overschedule, and emergencies do come up. Regardless of whether or not our slipups are avoidable (if avoidable—raising the possibility of a countertransference reaction), it is clearly an error to "atone" for our mistakes by overlooking similar mistakes in our patients. The patient's "mistake" or looseness about the rules either is unrelated to our own mistake (and hence relates only to what is going on inside of him), or is directly related to our behavior. In either case, it is important.

If, for example, patient lateness follows a session (or sessions) in which the group leader has been late, the group leader might raise this by saying, "I notice that several people have arrived late tonight (or over the past few weeks). I wonder how this might connect to my own lateness in recent weeks?" Alternatively, the therapist might simply note the lateness and ask what group members make of it. If group members respond with a litany of "legitimate" excuses, she might validate the reality that they present and wonder, in addition, how their being late (or at least their feelings about it) might relate to her own lateness at the last session (or during the past few weeks.)

Similarly, a therapist who occasionally makes billing errors (adding up the totals wrong, for example) may feel uncomfortable raising a patient's miscalculation on his payment check. But obviously, the same logic holds. Either the patient's behavior is directly linked to his perception of the therapist's carelessness and his feelings about it (in which case there is much to explore), or it is independent of the therapist's mistake (in which case there are equally useful paths to explore).

Handling Therapist Mistakes

It is obviously important that the therapist keep his mistakes to a minimum, and staying on top of countertransference reactions will carry him a long way toward achieving this goal. However, it is equally important, when mistakes do occur, that the therapist is sensitive to his patient's reactions about the mistakes and able to make the most of them therapeutically. Often small mistakes take on tremendous meaning for our patients.

> An extremely strong reaction occurred in one group when its leader accidentally ran the group 10 minutes overtime one evening. Given a 5-year history of great punctuality and precise time boundaries for ending each session, this deviation was quite noticeable. One member, wishing to protect the leader from perceived "fallibility," wondered if perhaps his watch had "lost time." Another speculated that the leader had done it on purpose in order to stimulate discussion (an explanation that this patient found preferable to the possibility that the leader had actually made a mistake). Other members tried to excuse the leader as "only human"—but, upon further exploration, were experiencing considerable discomfort about his "fallibility," which they associated with the unpredictability of their alcoholic parents.

As Winnicott (1955/1975) reminds us, "Failures there must be" (p. 298). However, the key to using these therapeutically is to understand that the therapist's present failure is "being used and must be treated as a past failure, one that the patient can perceive and encompass, and be angry about now." Winnicott explains the patient's intense anger over seemingly small therapist errors as a way of enabling the patient to be angry about past parental failures. The work of the therapist is, thus, to understand what was needed by the patient (and not forthcoming) at the time the original failure occurred.

Extricating Oneself from Erroneous Boundary Modifications

Occasionally, a group leader may be "caught off guard" and seduced into modifying a ground rule to his later regret. For example, in one of our newly formed groups, a member came in to her first session and announced that she would never be able to stay the entire hour and a half since her boss would not let her be away from work for so long. Under the pressure of the moment, the leader, while maintaining the importance of being in the group until the very end, offered the patient the option of coming 15–20 minutes late each week. Afterwards, when he had a chance to think about it, he regretted his decision but felt he would have to "live with his mistake." However, if a group leader rethinks one of his moves and feel that the position he has taken is untenable, it is important not only to understand how the error occurred, but also to feel that he can modify his position. Discussing the mistake with a colleague or supervisor who will help explore the countertransference pulls and pushes that led to the mistake will be helpful in avoiding similar mistakes in the future and providing perspective on how to modify the current error. For example, in the situation described, the leader was extremely anxious about the integrity of his group; it was a small group to begin with, and he was fearful about the prospect of losing the member if he stood firm about the ground rules—fears that were further exacerbated by having just joined the clinic and feeling that the success of this group was necessary to prove his competence as a group therapist.

Extrication from a mistake like the one above can be quite simple. After ascertaining that, indeed, a mistake has been made (by checking it out with a colleague), the leader can go in the next week and say, "I had some further thoughts about our discussion regarding Mary's arriving late each week. Perhaps others in the group did as well." He might then explore group members' thoughts and feelings about the issue and share his own thoughts as well, saying, "The more I thought about it, the more I felt that it wouldn't work." He might even share something of the dilemma that he was in at the time that he made the decision. Thus, he might say, "I was very much aware of wanting Mary to stay in the group and wanting it to be comfortable here for her, and I think that's what pulled me into considering the possibility of her arriving late each week. But the more I thought about it, the more I thought that while in the short run it might make Mary more comfortable, in the long-run, it would not be good for the group, and nobody (including Mary) would be able to get as much work done here".

If the group tries to nail the leader on the fact that he made a mistake (saying something like, "Well, how come you weren't thinking about that last week?" or, "So, are you telling us that you made a mistake?"), it is important that the leader explore with the group how it feels to have had the leader make a mistake. As indicated earlier, group members may have tremendously complicated feelings about a leader's mistake. Particularly in the beginning, when much of the initial glue that keeps patients in therapy has to do with positive transference, idealization, and unrealistic fantasies about the therapist —acknowledging that the leader can be fallible takes on considerable importance. Thus, if a mistake is made, I might say, "How does it feel to know that your leader has made a mistake?" This question acknowledges that a mistake has been made—but, more important than the confession, pushes the group to explore how they feel about this.

Seeking Consultation or Supervision When You Want to Bend a Rule

Mistakes, although not entirely avoidable, can be kept to a minimum by seeking consultation or supervision whenever you are considering doing something different with your group or with an individual member of the group that reflects a deviation from your general operating ground rules. But what kind of supervision or assistance should you seek out? Therapists are sometimes inclined to ask for "consultation" from somebody who they think is likely to support what they want to do—a colleague who they know is "flexible" in the particular area in which they are considering making a change. It is probably a good idea, instead, to pick a colleague or supervisor who you suspect is likely to be a little bit more conservative than you are—someone who may challenge you to think more about what you are doing rather than simply giving you a green light. In this regard, I am reminded of the story of the sinner who had catalogued all of the confessionals in town and knew which priests were light on which sins. When he felt he needed to confess, he would pick a church accordingly. While he thus accomplished one of his goals (expiation), the real purpose of seeking out a wise superior was lost.

Choosing between Supervision and Psychotherapy

I have highlighted the importance of the therapist's ability to stay on top of countertransference reactions and, in general, to be appropriately self-aware and reflective about the course of the therapy and his work with the patient. Supervision—whether with peers or with a senior therapist, individually or in a supervision group—can be very helpful for this purpose. Supervision provides a rich arena, not only for processing and sorting out what is going on in the group, but also for exploring countertransference feelings—both objective and subjective—that will contribute substantially to the quality and depth of your clinical work.

At times, particularly when countertransference feelings are intense, there may be a temptation on the part of either supervisor or supervisee to blur the boundaries between supervision and psychotherapy. However, as Kanfer and Schefft (1988) clearly state, "both supervisor and student must be careful not to violate the structure and purpose of supervision" (p. 370). The focus of the work in a supervisory hour should be on understanding what is going on in the therapist, as a way of better understanding the dynamics of her patients and of her group. When the therapists' own conflicts need addressing, therapy, in addition to supervision, should be sought.

Although the case for returning to psychotherapy, in conjunction with (or instead of) supervision, cannot be simply stated, there are a few useful guidelines. Psychotherapy might be indicated if countertransference slippage around rules and expectations seems to be occurring with many of your patients. Often this is accompanied by a feeling of being "out of control" and "stirred up" by your work. (You may notice that you are spending more and more time worrying about your patients—or about your own behavior with them.) Another signpost that therapy may be indicated is finding yourself, as you listen to your patients, slipping into thoughts about your own past, or about your own present difficulties. When this occurs, it is apparent that the patient's material is triggering so much inside of you that it becomes difficult for you to stay with the patient.

Occasionally, senior therapists who have been in psychotherapy earlier in their careers react to the idea of returning to therapy by feeling that this implies that they have "regressed" in some way. I believe that this is rarely the case. All of us continue to rework important issues from the past throughout our lives. With each new stage of our own development, as we take on new patient populations, as we try out new kinds of professional activities, we have an opportunity to rework important issues from the past.

Personal Issues in the Life of the Therapist

The therapist's own personal life experiences and conflicts may cause further countertransference roadblocks. It is likely the the therapist's personal life experiences and conflicts will resonate along a number of dimensions with those of the patients that he treats. As Kanfer and Schefft (1988) point out, it is important for the therapist to be aware of sensitive or unsettled personal areas and to pay special attention when working with patients who are struggling with similar issues. For example, a therapist who has recently succeeded in getting his alcoholic wife into treatment may need to pay special attention to his reactions to a patient whose alcoholic partner is still abusively drinking. Therapists who are themselves recovering from substance abuse may be particularly vulnerable to powerful reactions when group members repeatedly relapse. Similarly, a therapist who is recently divorced or separated may need to exercise special caution in treating patients whose central presenting issue involves marital discord.

When working with patients whose issues resonate with the therapist's, blurring of boundaries is more likely. It is thus important that the therapist is clear about the ground rules and, when one of them is about to be broken, that he makes a conscious and thoughtful decision that such a modification is in the patient's best interest. When rules are broken without any active decision on the part of the therapist, we can usually infer that countertransference issues are being stirred up—and that the therapist's behavior may not, in fact, be in the patient's best interest (Langs, 1975). The therapist concerned about the impact of his own personal issues on his clinical work may need to seek out additional support or consultation (through personal therapy or supervision). If complications remain and the therapist continues to feel that her own reactions are getting in the way of a particular patient's therapeutic growth, referral to another therapist should be considered. (See Vannicelli, 1989, for a fuller discussion of these issues.)

In addition to specific unresolved issues in the life of the therapist that may complicate or impede his ability to help his patients with their journeys, it is likely that the therapist's development and level of integration, more generally, imposes a ceiling on the level of development that will be reached by the group as a whole or by individual members within the group.* As is often the case in families when offspring surpass the accomplishments of their parents, anxiety is produced in group members if an individual member or the group as a whole moves beyond the level of development of the leader. Even if the group has the potential to do this and begins to move ahead, regression ultimately is likely. Although it is important to consider the possibility that the therapist can also grow along with the group, it is in fact the therapist's responsibility to take care of his own growth in another arena (i.e., in his own psychotherapy).

We understand more clearly how the leader's own issues can hold back the group when we consider a clinical example such as the following, in which an ACOA therapist's unresolved issues caused her to collude with the group's resistance.

This ACOA group, during the first few weeks of its formation, struggled to identify the "most problematic patient." The leader found herself, by the end of the first session, colluding with the group—feeling, with them, that a particular "problem patient" did not "fit" in the group and allowing the group to persuade this member that he did not belong. When the patient did not return the following week, the leader expressed relief, stating in supervision "the group would be better off without this patient, who really was too sick." The leader's own wish to "save the family" by "ridding it of its troubled member"—a dynamic that she was all too familiar with her own family of origin—blinded her to the realization of what the group (and she) was reenacting. Instead, she colluded with them and helped this "unfit" patient leave the group, thus recapitulating the

---

*A theory put forth by Allen Surkis in a workshop, "The Group Therapist's Quandary: To Lead or to Treat." Presented at 10th International Congress on Group Psychotherapy, Amsterdam, 1989.

family fantasy that everything would be fine if only the problem member were removed. A few weeks later the group took up the same cause again, searching anew for a problem patient to eliminate. At this point, the leader, understanding her own earlier collusion, was able to intervene more effectively and this time helped the group retain and work with the new problem patient that it had identified.

THE LEADER'S ROLE AND CLINICAL STANCE

The group leader is like the conductor of an orchestra—fine-tuning each part and helping the many voices to clearly articulate as well as to integrate with one another. The experienced conductor, baton in hand, knows his place and knows what he needs to do in order to create the integrated experience that he is hoping for. More simply put, he knows where he stands in relationship to the orchestra. A major roadblock for many group leaders is not having a clear idea about where they stand in relationship to their groups. Successful leader roles from other nonclinical situations tug for expression (teacher, scout leader, committee chair), as do therapist's behaviors appropriate for use in individual therapy. But how does the leader know how to choose the appropriate responses from this repertoire of related behaviors? Clearly, in dynamically oriented interactional therapy groups, simply applying one's repertoire of responses from individual therapy is not adequate. Group therapy is not simply individual therapy within a group. But what about those other leader functions that are so well ingrained from other situations? Which of those are appropriate? And how does he differentiate those functions the group can do for itself from those that he has to provide?

Although I tend to use the words group "therapist" and group "leader" somewhat interchangeably, Allen Surkis* has delineated some useful distinctions between the leader and the therapist functions—both of which are important throughout the life of the group, but differentially so based on phase of group development. Surkis maintains that leadership functions take precedence over therapy functions, since the former are necessary to dilute the group's anxiety and animate the group so that it can effectively do the work of therapy.

---

*Allen Surkis. "The Group Therapist's Quandary: To Lead or to Treat." Workshop presented at 10th International Congress of Group Psychotherapy, Amsterdam, 1989.

Thus, leadership functions predominate in the early stages of group life, and as time goes on, the therapist functions become more important. Leadership functions are also necessary: (1) to help the group get past resistances (either in the form of an interpretation or in helping the group bypass resistance); (2) when boundary issues are being violated (restating the group goals and exploring the group's slippage); and (3) when emotions are so intense that they "interfere with reason." As Surkis points out, when a new patient enters the group, leader functions may again temporarily predominate (unless the group itself is able to provide this function—letting the new member know what to expect and how the group works).

In contrast, the therapist or "treating" functions that Surkis describes include the following: (1) promoting a sense of discovery, (2) attempting to provide a corrective emotional experience, and (3) helping patients to get in touch with themselves and to reintegrate parts that have been closed off. As he points out, in order to do the therapeutic tasks, trust must be established in the group (reinforced by the leader functions) along with the basic sense that others are good and caring. As the group evolves, both the leader and the therapist functions become less important, as group members learn how to "co-lead" and to assume some of these functions with one another.

A major roadblock for many group therapists is an inability to differentiate those functions that the group can do for itself from those that need to be provided by the leader. This is often experienced by the leader as confusion about how active to be. More correctly stated, the question should be in what ways to be active. The issue is not how much to say, but what to say and when to say it (and when to refrain from doing so). Clearly, there are certain functions that the leader has to provide for the group until the group can provide for itself—in particular, tasks related to helping the group look at itself and how it operates, which, in the beginning, a group is not likely to even think about doing for itself. Group members (like group leaders) initially bring to bear many prior kinds of group experiences that may be very different from the kind of behavior that is called for in a therapy group, e.g., experiences in Al-Anon or AA, where processing group interaction is not the important thing, but telling one's story is (along with possible feedback and advice). It is not that group members come in with bad intentions about how to behave, but often prior learnings compete with the kinds of behaviors most useful for growth in a therapy group. Members must learn how a group works—a function that the leader initially has to help with (as exemplified by some of the leader interventions discussed in Chapter 4).

Pursuing difficult topics or impasses in the group also initially falls to the leader when group members do not know how to perform this function for themselves or for the group. It is important for the group leader to speak up when something needs to be said that the group may not be able to get to, or when something needs to be examined that will not happen unless the leader intervenes. If the group can make such an intervention for itself—for example, can ask for more information about something, can express confusion, can provide empathic responses—there is no reason for the leader to do so. The leader should perform only nonredundant functions (those that are not already in the repertoire of the group), role modeling new behaviors that eventually the group members can take on and perform for themselves.

It is important for group leaders to understand that the issue is more "what you do when you are active" than "how active you are." It is important to be fairly active in (1) helping the group stay focused on the process, (2) undercutting boredom (by interpreting resistance and examining conflict in the room that creates a "stuck" feeling), and (3) helping the group look at the "misses" (e.g., when something important has happened that has been ignored by the group). If the group leader is process oriented, she is less concerned with keeping the material flowing (the group can generally do this) than with processing the interruptions in the flow and in helping the group understand its defenses. Thus, when I ask the group to notice what has just happened (usually when there is some kind of interruption in the flow, or when a patient has not been responded to), I do so not just to "get back on track." Rather, I do so because I think that the "bypass" action is itself important and to be understood—reflecting an important group process and the kinds of defenses that are used individually and collectively when group members become anxious or uncomfortable. This is valuable information for a group in which members are engaged in understanding themselves—how they operate as individuals and how the group as a whole operates.

After a while, the group will also come to recognize its own defensive functions—for example, that people change the subject as a rescue operation if they feel that others are on the "hot seat," and especially if they have resonating anxiety when the topic is "too close to home." Members will also learn shorthand ways of referring to this. They will thus monitor their own functioning by saying things like, "Was that a rescue operation, Bill?" or, "Is it getting too hot in the kitchen?" The group will learn how to perform these functions once they understand that these are the kind of defensive operations that people use to deal with uncomfortable situations. They will be guided initially by the leader's questions such as, "I wonder if you wanted to rescue Carol just then?" or, "I wonder if there is something in this that was stirring up some feelings in you that were a little uncomfortable?" The empathic response communicates understanding to the interrupter as well as to the person who has been interrupted. It says, I have a feeling there was something important going on for you just then, and I am interested in that, as well.

Often leaders are paying careful attention to the process but neglect to ask about it when something is not being addressed. It is not that they have not noticed, but that they are reluctant to ask a question about it unless they already know the answer. But it is not necessary for you to fully understand the situation when you ask a question; all that is important is that you have registered that there is something going on that doesn't seem to fit—or that something important seems to have been missed. Since group members usually assume that when you ask a question you do know the answer, if you are queried about this, you can respond, "I'm not quite sure, but it seems like something is going on that we may want to pay a little more attention to." Or you may comment, "This sort of thing has happened in here before. What do you suppose it tells us about the way this group operates?" The leader's questions repeatedly point to the fact that there is something understandable in the process—even when it seems amiss. We simply need to come to understand it.

One category of therapist activity that can usually be reduced (particularly in the beginning therapist who is prone to excesses in this area) is information gathering, since this is something that group members are usually perfectly good at doing for themselves. But the group will need the leader's help if it is to learn how not to be just a series of people who come in weekly to report, but rather, an effective group of people who can genuinely engage and interact with one another. Another category of activity that most beginning therapists can considerably diminish is "conversational" or keeping the flow going. Often leaders feel anxious when there are silences and feel that they must provide conversational cement (perhaps with informational questioning). Instead, it is far more useful for leaders to process with the group what is going on, what the silences are about, and what their expectations are of the leader and of the other members in relationship to the group's task. It is important that a group leader ask only those questions that he feels the group members cannot ask—doing only what the group needs him to do. The leader's job is either to perform the needed functions for the group (more necessary in initial sessions) or to process with the group how it is that the group is not performing those functions itself.

The Didactic Mode

Keeping in mind that the task of the leader is to help the group process and explore, it may also be useful for us to consider again the difference between a dynamically oriented therapy group and an education group. Although both experiences are educative in nature, the goal of the therapy group is not specifically to provide information or to evaluate members' behaviors. In a therapy group, the goal is to help patients process each member's experiences and ongoing events within the group. Although gathering of information and receiving evaluative feedback will occur within the context of the therapy group, the goal is to help patients learn to do this for themselves and for one another in the group.

Particularly when the group is stuck, anxious, or seems to be in need of leader assistance, leaders are often tempted to step into the "teacher mode," more appropriate for an education group or classroom situation. This is understandable, since the classroom is the most familiar group context for both members and leaders, and at times of stress leaders may fall back on their many years of classroom experience. The other didactic mode that leaders sometimes fall into during stressful periods in the group is the "mother role"—again understandably regressing to the familiar "fix-it" position with which we have all had a great deal of experience (either as the recipient or as the fixer). However, as Winnicott (1965) admonishes, emphasizing the importance of the therapist remaining "professionally involved," the therapist "is not a rescuer, a teacher, an ally, or a moralist" (p.

162). Mother/teacher-tone questions (as differentiated from questions that encourage the patient to process for herself what is going on) might include: "Susan, do you think that is really a good idea?" or, a statement such as, "What you need to do is . . . ." A more neutral position that alerts the patient to consider and reflect upon her options might be expressed by commenting: "What thoughts did you have about how that might work for you?" "Has it worked out in the past?" or, "What would it be like for you if you did do such and such?" What distinguishes the therapist/leader mode from the mother/teacher mode is that questions and statements are framed in such a way as to leave the patient in a position to continue to process her experience; the patient is encouraged to continue to explore what her options are, and what various choices might mean to her.

The Closed-Ended Question

When the leader wishes to more fully explore feelings, thoughts, and fantasies, it is useful to avoid questions that simply lead to yes/no answers and to phrase questions, instead, in a way that will lead to fuller responses. In general, questions that begin with "how" or "in what way" are more useful for this purpose than questions that begin with "why" or "do you" or "are you," which are more likely to lead to simple yes/no answers.

Although asking questions is an important part of the group leader's task, patients often comment that they feel "put on the spot" by therapists' questions. They reexperience the anxiety of the classroom, feeling that a particular answer is expected and that they must produce what they imagine their therapist is looking for. Though to some extent this is inevitable (and, itself, an issue to be explored), questions can often be rendered more palatable if they have an open, invitational style that conveys genuine curiosity and interest.

It should be noted that exploration of process and promotion of self-evaluation through a curious/questioning style, while important, may need to be temporarily abridged or abandoned when a patient actively poses a threat to herself or others. Under such circumstances, it is often essential for the therapist to assume "a highly directive role, taking charge of the treatment situation" (Kanfer & Schefft, 1988, p.

353) and giving specific feedback (and evaluation) to the patient involved, along with clearly stated recommendations or plans for protecting the patient against her destructive impulses.

Obfuscating by Being Too Quick

Although it goes without saying that as therapists we aim to communicate clearly with our patients, there are times when the message may be more effectively delivered by something less than our most clever and precise articulation. Epstein (1979) alludes to this, stating:

> . . . I find that it sometimes helps matters if the patient has the feeling that I may not be having the easiest time in understanding him. . . . What this does is create a more favorable distribution of good and bad parts and of power. All badness and inferiority is no longer all within the patient; nor is all goodness and superiority within me. He feels more comfortable with me as a person who is more like himself. (pp. 268-269)

In a similar vein, a favorite mentor of mine, Alfred Stanton, used to say, "The perfect interpretation is not one which stuns the patient with our brilliance (and possibly humiliates him into wondering why he hadn't thought of it) but one which gently and slowly is spun out with the patient." He used to point out that his best interpretations were those that he stuttered out in clumsy fashion with the help of his patient, who chewed on them, clarified them, and presented them back in metabolized form. In group therapy, too, I often find it useful to stumble through important interpretations, using my own confusion (and the need to get the matter sorted out) as a technique. When I feel this will be useful, I am likely to present my thoughts quite loosely, and often haltingly, encouraging group members' active involvement in clarifying and refining.

There are also times when I make what I think is a clear statement or interpretation which leads to a confused reaction on the part of the patient, who has been unable to "digest" what I have put forth. I generally respond to the patient's confusion with a comment such as, "I don't think I've put that very clearly" or "That really was kind of confusing, wasn't it?" I then engage other members of the group in trying to sort out what it was that I was trying to say and to say it "better" for me.

Therapeutic, Nontherapeutic, and Antitherapeutic Responses

Throughout these pages I have attempted to describe a leader's stance that maximizes the occurrence of therapeutic interventions and minimizes the occurrence of nontherapeutic and antitherapeutic interventions. The difference between the latter two is that a nontherapeutic response is not particularly useful and may serve as "noise." Like chitchat, it is similar to the kind of social response that might occur outside of the therapy context and does little to specifically further the therapeutic work. In contrast, antitherapeutic responses (usually motivated by unexplored countertransference) are therapist responses that actually interfere with the effectiveness of the therapeutic work. Although one might argue that even nontherapeutic responses in some way may interfere, since they might either dilute the transference or possibly confuse some of what is transpiring, I differentiate them from antitherapeutic responses, which clearly interfere with the work and may seriously jeopardize the success of the therapeutic venture.

It may be helpful to think of therapeutic responses as those that are directly responsive to the work that the patient needs to do—that respond in a relevant way to the patient's issues and to his transference reactions as they unfold in the therapeutic relationship. Nontherapeutic responses, on the other hand, have little to do with the therapeutic task. And antitherapeutic responses are generally those that occur as undisciplined responses to countertransference reactions in the therapist. The most disciplined therapists have very high ratios of therapeutic responses compared to the other two categories of response. Less disciplined therapists may weave in more nontherapeutic responses, and unskilled therapist (and those caught up in serious countertransference reactions) may actually behave antitherapeutically. Experience helps in shifting the balance toward therapeutic responses on the part of the group leader, but experience is no substitute for training and good supervision.

Therapist Self-Disclosure and Affect Transparency

One of the most confusing dilemmas for therapists—and perhaps for group therapists in particular (and also one of the most hotly debated areas in the group psychotherapy literature)—relates to the therapist's transparency about his thoughts, feelings, and personal information about himself. As Dies (1983) points out:

> The research literature on therapist self-disclosure is inconclusive in demonstrating uniform effects of "transparency." Some investigators offer positive conclusions (e.g., Dies et al., 1979; Hurley and Force, 1973), others report that therapist self-disclosure is unimportant (e.g., Bolman, 1971, 1973), while still others find that self-disclosure may even be detrimental (e.g., Lieberman et al., 1973). In the final analysis perhaps all of these researchers are correct; the effect of therapist self-disclosure depends more precisely on such variables as the type of group, stage of group development, and the content of the disclosure itself. (p. 40)

Ultimately, each therapist will find his own way in this regard and hopefully will develop a consistent position that guides him beyond the neophyte's position of "just doing whatever feels right at the moment" or "just being honest." The position that I take of minimal self-disclosure and transparency is consistent with the writings of many psychodynamically oriented group therapists (Cooper, 1988; Rutan & Stone, 1984; West & Livesley, 1986) as well as cognitive behavior therapists (Kanfer & Schefft, 1988). It is not simply the stance of a "withholding" therapist, since (as the reader will have discerned through the many interventions that I have described) I am by no means an inactive therapist. I talk when I feel it will be useful (perhaps sometimes more than I should), and I say those things that I feel will help further the work. However, when it comes to questions about personal issues in my own life and facts about myself, or questions about my feelings, I have generally found in my own work and in the work of the many therapists that I have supervised that there are usually productive (and, in my opinion, preferable) alternatives to self-disclosure. As Dies (1983) points out,

> Self-disclosure is only one of many possible interventions available to the group leader, however, and like most other interventions, its effectiveness will undoubtedly depend on the extent to which it is systematically integrated into a more comprehensive model of group leadership. Therapist transparency can encourage corresponding behavior among group members, yet we also know that even without sharing feelings and experiences, therapists can generate self-revelation within the group. (p. 42)

The Rationale for Not Answering Direct Questions or Providing Personal Information about Oneself

As I have indicated, I generally do not answer direct personal questions and rarely volunteer personal information about myself—either spontaneously or when asked directly. My rationale for both of these "withholding" positions is that I am making every attempt to clearly differentiate the discourse and process of therapy from routine social exchange. And I believe that this differentiation is particularly important within the defined parameters of the therapeutic hour, as well as entering and leaving the sessions. Thus, when a patient says at the beginning of the hour, "How are you?" I would avoid saying, "Fine, thank you, how are you?" Instead, I might say simply "OK" or simply smile or nod to acknowledge that I have heard the question and wait for the material to unfold. Or, if the patient's "How are you?" is out of character for her, I might ask if she had particular concerns this session about how I might be. Similarly, if a patient sits down and a few minutes after beginning the session says, "That's a really pretty dress," I would consider this part of the therapeutic material and make a mental note about it (even if I did not, at that point, comment on it). In a similar vein, if the patient interrupted what she was saying to comment on how I looked, I might ask, "What was happening just then?"

My assumption, clearly communicated by my behavior, is that everything that happens within the therapy hour is to be understood as material that is relevant to our work together. My behavior clearly indicates that nothing that we are doing is simply social banter or casual pleasant social exchange. I do not take this position because I enjoy it—in fact, it would often be preferable to be able to kibitz with my patients. I behave the way I do because I think it maximizes the opportunity for us to effectively use the limited time that we have together.

Sometimes I am asked by trainees, "Would you behave the same way at the drinking fountain 20 minutes before the session?" Although I would not do a total turnabout at the drinking fountain—spontaneously volunteering "what a hard day it's been" or any other personal information about myself, I would treat an exchange at the drinking fountain in a manner that moves slightly more toward a social exchange. There, if the patient said, "Hi Dr. Vannicelli, how're you doing!" I might respond "Good, thank you." A comment about the weather would also be responded to. If the patient says "It's quite a scorcher isn't it?" I might respond "I don't remember when we had such a hot August." A comment about a nice dress at the drinking fountain would be responded to by saying "Thank you." I would make no attempts to process material at that time, but if it seemed as if the material was important, I might store it up for consideration in a later therapeutic context. Alternatively, if the behavior seemed to be totally in keeping with natural social exchange, in a circumstance in which natural social exchange would be called for, I would not be inclined to use it further.

It is of some interest that therapists are almost universally more comfortable self-disclosing about aspects of themselves that they are pleased with (or that they think their patients will approve of) than about less appealing aspects of themselves. Thus, even the self-disclosing therapist is more likely to answer some questions than others. However, it is essential that the therapist fully understand what is motivating her stance with regard to answering direct personal questions. For example, a therapist is asked as she departs for her vacation, "Where are you going?" she responds, "To the east coast." The patient then gets braver, "Oh, are you going with your family?" Here the therapist realizes that things are escalating and simply smiles and says "I'll see you in 2 weeks." Clearly the message that has been given is that although some questions may be answered, there is a limit to which the personal boundaries will be extended. This is OK—to a lesser or a greater degree all of us answer some questions and don't answer others. But let us consider now the issue of consistency. What if the next time the therapist is taking a vacation, her life is a mess, and now, on the eve of her week's scheduled vacation, she has absolutely no plans. She is simply planning to "veg out." Now, how will she respond to the question, "where are you going? She is unlikely to say, "I have no plans." Similarly, to the question "Are you married?" therapists who are married may feel relatively comfortable saying "Yes." But what if they are not? Or what if they are currently going through a divorce? Then how do they answer? I am sometimes asked whether I don't think all this is "grist for the mill" that could be processed. Indeed I do, but my own view is that while there may be ample opportunity, particularly in individual therapy, to process all of this, in a group where there are seven or eight people who may each be affected differently by the therapist's disclosure, these self-disclosures generally add unnecessary clutter that is not particularly useful to the therapy.

I am also sometimes asked, "What if one therapist thinks it's OK to answer these questions in the group and the other co-therapist does not?" My response to this is that the two therapists should work out a single position that they are both comfortable with. Otherwise, the therapist who does not answer questions is perceived as cold and responding without any therapeutic rationale for her withholding behavior, and group members (who generally would feel more gratified to have at least some questions answered) will be in alliance with the "nonwithholding" therapist.

This kind of situation also comes up frequently in substance-abuse programs, where some members of the staff are recovering and others are not. My own view is that it is useful that there be a consistent position taken by the staff. The position might be that questions about whether or not they are recovering will be explored, and an answer given ("yes" or "no"), if, after exploration, it seems clinically useful to do so. Or the position may be that none of the therapists directly answer this question. Or a reasonable position may be that the question is always simply routinely answered. For those who are recovering to simply answer, and those who are not to explore or withhold, strikes me as an odd position that is difficult to justify clinically.

Does all this mean that I never answer a question directly or ever give information about myself? No. But when I do, I have (hopefully) thought about it carefully, and I have a clear reason for believing that, in this instance, providing the information will be more useful than withholding it. Let me give an example of a situation in which it seemed to me and my co-leader that some personal information would be helpful to our group, despite the fact that it was uncharacteristic for us to do so.

I had been out of work for several weeks with back problems, just following termination of the co-therapist with whom I had worked for 8 years. A substitute leader had covered the group during this time, who then joined me as the new co-leader. Two weeks after I returned, he needed to announce to the group that he would be gone for 3 weeks (for his wedding and honeymoon). Because the timing was clearly out of keeping with what we felt would have been appropriate care and concern for the group, we decided that in this instance it would be useful to say to the group, "Clearly it is not very good timing, in terms of all that has been going on here, for Dr. A to be away for 3 weeks. Had we been able to work it in any other way we would have, but his wedding and honeymoon were planned long before all this began." (It should be noted that while I can also imagine not providing this information, after much discussion and consideration it was our decision that providing it, in this instance, would be more useful than not.)

Similarly, a colleague of mine got a call early in the morning about the death of a very close friend. She was extremely shaken and, had there been time, would have canceled her morning sessions that day. Her first patient arrived moments later. Since it was clear that something was amiss, the therapist appropriately decided that the patient needed to be told something—even though it was personal—about what was going on with the therapist. Thus, she said, "I learned just a little while ago that a dear friend has just died. I am not quite myself this morning, but I will listen as best I can." If the therapist actually felt that she could not listen, it would have been appropriate for her (or her secretary) to tell the patient what had happened, explain that she didn't think that she would be able to give the patient the attention that he deserved, and reschedule the session.

Self-Disclosure Dilemmas around Personal Credentials

Often the demands for self-disclosure that therapists feel the most conflicted about are requests for information about personal aspects of their lives that seem to bear directly on the presenting issue that their patients wish to work on, (for example, in an ACOA group, the question of whether the therapist is herself an ACOA; in a recovery group, whether the therapist is recovering; in a couples group, whether the therapist is herself married or coupled). Yet, other questions are often equally important to the patient—for example, how experienced is the therapist? It is important to recognize that simple, "straightforward" responses may not, in fact, be responsive to the concerns that are being raised by such questions. What is generally being raised is a wish for reassurance that the therapist will have the appropriate credentials to help the patient with his areas of concern.

Let us examine, for example, the question to the couples therapist, "Are you married?" Though not stated, what is generally of interest in such a question is not simply whether or not the therapist is married, but whether her personal experience has been adequate to effectively deal with the relationship problems that the patient presents. (A successful marriage might well be a credential—but would 10 years of strained, impoverished relating, even if one were still with the same partner?) Since in most instances what the patient is requesting is reassurance that the therapist will be able to help, what is most important in handling these questions is not the precise answer that is given—or even whether or not a specific answer is given—but how the question is handled. In general, I have found that when therapists are uncomfortable with a question (often because the patient's doubts resonate with their own), they either rush in too quickly to answer or in some way convey defensiveness. These responses are generally motivated by resonating countertransference feelings in the therapist—that is, her own concerns about her level of expertise, credentials, and ability, ultimately, to help.

The following clinical vignette illustrates this situation.

> Not long ago, a new group leader in our clinic who had just gotten his Ph.D. was "initiated" his first night in the group with the question, "What degree do you have?" The new young leader, instead of merely stating that he had a Ph.D. in psychology, was so anxious that he gave a full educational history citing the school and year in which all of his degrees were confirmed—his two masters degrees, his B.A., going all the way back to high school! Although the young therapist's response may not have felt quite as reassuring as he had hoped, what was more important was that he had shown his lack of expertise by hastily answering the question without doing anything to process its underlying meaning.

As this example illustrates, patients often need reassurance about the therapist's skill and ability to handle problems in areas that are also conflictual for the therapist. Understanding what the questions trigger in the therapist is essential to adequate handling of the patient's concerns. As this example also illustrates, pressures toward therapist self-disclosure are often particularly intense at the beginning of the group venture—when either a member or leader has just entered the group. This is a natural part of figuring out something about the rules and boundaries in the group, as well as the patient's way of ascertaining whether the therapist will be able to help.

It should be noted that a simple, "straightforward" response may convince the patient that she cannot get the kind of help that she needs. For example, for the recovering substance abuser, the leader's response, "No, I am not 'in recovery,'" may leave the patient feeling, "How can you possibly understand what I have been through when you have no idea what it's like to give up alcohol or drugs?" Even the response, "I too am an alcoholic," may be a double-edged sword. While for some patients this may initially seem like the only acceptable answer, for others it may signal that the therapist is "no better off than we are" and "not equipped to care for us."

In all likelihood, the reason that this question is frequently handled as if there is nothing more to it than simple curiosity is that many therapists are persuaded by the success of the many alcohol-related self-help groups (AA, Al-Anon, and Al-Anon/ACOA groups), where, indeed, all help is provided by others with similar problems. Thus, the therapist who would ordinarily explore or interpret similar questions from other patients (e.g., from a mother who wants to know if the therapist has trouble with her adolescents) may neglect to explore requests about drinking status from recovering patients or requests from ACOAs regarding the therapist's family of origin. However, it is essential to interpret for the substance abuser or ACOA, as it would be in the parallel instance for other patients, the concerns underlying these questions about the therapist.

A related self-disclosure hazard for therapists who are in a 12-step program is that they may find themselves pulled toward the "self-help" model with concomitant pressures toward self-disclosure and sharing of personal experiences (as one might do in the role of an AA or Al-Anon sponsor). For such therapists, at times it may be confusing how the role of therapist differs from or converges upon that of sponsor. But it is essential to recognize that the two roles are quite different. A sponsor continues to help himself while also helping the other. While in the course of our work, we as therapists also continue to grow, our growth is never the focus of the therapeutic relationship; it is always the patient's growth that comes first.

I have found it useful in my own practice to have a basic policy about self-disclosure which I explain to patients whenever personal questions come up. What I generally say to patients when they ask a personal question about me is the following: "Generally, I do not find it useful to share personal information about myself. However, I'd be interested in knowing more about how this particular question might be important to you, and how a given answer of one sort or another might be useful." Implicit in my statement is a suggestion that together, the patient and I will consider whether a modification in my policy might be useful in this particular instance. I generally find that patients are comforted by the knowledge that I am willing to explore the issue, and perhaps comforted most of all by understanding that there are thoughtful ground rules guiding my work. Almost inevitably, these discussions eventuate in a clarification of the patient's concerns about whether I will be able to understand and help with the important work that she has come to tackle.

Alternative to Self-Disclosure for Sharing Personal Experience

Sometimes a therapist may feel that some aspect of her own personal experience might be of value to the patient. However, if she shares the material directly, the message that she hopes to communicate may be complicated by the patient's response to the personal information that she has just learned about the therapist. An alternative to self-disclosure that avoids this complication is to provide the information via a vignette about someone else—"a woman that I work with," "a young woman that I know quite well," etc. Instead of saying to a patient who is being taken to court by her ex-husband, "When I found myself in a similar situation a few years ago, I found myself feeling . . .," I might say, "When a friend of mine was in a similar situation, she found herself feeling conflicted—on the one hand wanting to take care of herself but, on the other hand, concerned about having to publicly confront somebody that she cared about." In this way, the same material can be shared, without creating a situation in which the patient has to simultaneously deal with the transferential implications of the new piece of personal information that she has just learned about the therapist.

Self-Disclosure about Feelings

Up to now we have been talking primarily about self-disclosure regarding factual personal information about the therapist. There are many group therapists (even among those who are relatively conservative about disclosing factual information about themselves) who believe that self-disclosure about their feelings is helpful to the group in role modeling open communication, honesty, and sharing of feelings. Sometimes a therapist's self-disclosure can be helpful in making group members feel safe to disclose their own feelings. However, while therapist's self-disclosure of feelings can be helpful, the research literature also indicates that, at times, it can actually be harmful (Lieberman et al., 1973; Weigel, Dinges, Dyer, & Straumfjord, 1972). Simply role modeling "honesty" is apparently not the answer, since as Dies and Cohen (1976) found from content analysis of therapist self-disclosures, patients reacted very differently to positive therapist disclosures (sharing positive strivings and normal emotional experiences such as sadness or anxiety) than to negative therapist disclosure (such as angrily confronting individual members or criticizing the group by disclosing feelings of frustration or boredom). Particularly for the beginning therapist, the task of determining which of his "honest feelings" to share, and which to hold back, may pose a nearly insurmountable challenge. He cannot "just trust his gut," nor can he just act as he might were he himself a member of the group.

Although I do not disagree that in the hands of a skilled group therapist thoughtful self-disclosure of the therapist's feelings may, at times, be useful, I believe that in most instances, the skilled leader will be able to help the group move from one place to another without disclosing her own feelings; and that modeling of empathy, ways of expressing feelings, and ways of communicating are done in many different ways in our work as leaders. As group leaders we model much more than listening—we model empathic attunement with our faces. Moreover, through our comments and questions, we underscore the large range of feelings that are possible and help patients understand that they may be experiencing conflictual feelings. I tend to be cautious and conservative about self-disclosure regarding my own feelings, particularly in a group, because I think that it is important to know, when making a self-disclosure, how it will be understood by the listener and what therapeutic impact it will have. Although at times this is difficult to know, even in individual therapy, it is approximately eightfold harder in a group, where the therapist's sensitivities must be on the pulse of eight people, not just one. This is not to say that I do not use any kind of self-disclosure. There are, in fact, a few categories of affectual self-disclosure that I do use from time to time.

One such self-disclosure is to share the fact that I am feeling in conflict—stating that I am worried that if I move in one direction, such and such will happen, but if I fail to move, something else equally troublesome might occur. Or I might share that I am worried that if we let this issue drop, Mary may feel as if we don't care, but if we continue to pursue her, she will feel as if we are on the attack (here my own worry is self-disclosed). Clearly, these kinds of self-disclosures about my feelings are in the interest of describing my relationship to the group process and guiding subsequent group transactions.

Other self-disclosures that I make may at times take the form of a "we" statement that includes myself—for example, "My guess is that everybody in here has had important losses." Or, "I think its going to be hard for all of us to say good-bye to Maryanne."

The most complicated self-disclosures that I share make use of projective identification. In this kind of disclosure, after I have fully examined my own feelings in reaction to the patient and have come to understand the part of these feelings that corresponds to what the patient experiences in his inner world, I disclose how I am feeling as a way of connecting to what I think is going on for him. Thus, I describe the feelings that are induced in me (the self-disclosure) as a way of helping the patient know that I do, indeed, understand. I usually think such self-disclosures out carefully before I say them— even sometimes writing them out in advance for myself to be sure that they are clear. The following vignette illustrates the use of this kind of self-disclosure.

> While working with Mr. W, I increasingly found myself conflicted about making the wrong response and discomforted by the prospect that I would be chided by him for missing the point whichever way I turned. If I supported his strengths I would be criticized for not seeing how bad and dysfunctional he was; if I allied with his eternal feelings that something was the matter with him, I would be seen as critical and missing his strengths. Using my own countertransference feelings I ultimately said, "I think I understand something of the dilemma that you have felt. Lately, particularly at times when you have been feeling especially bad about yourself and perhaps even worried that you might be coming unglued, I felt myself conflicted about where I might stand that could be of use to you—feeling that if I sided with the part of you that felt bad, damaged, and as if you were crumbling, that while in some ways you might feel understood, in other ways you would see me as your critical, disparaging mother who saw you as a bad and damaged person. On the other hand, I have felt that if I sided with your strength and hope, you might in some ways perceive this as a positive message, but you might also feel as if I was invalidating your mother (and the important part of her that lives inside of you). I think this conflict about where to stand lives in you as well. To see yourself as healthy feels like a repudiation of your mother (and, ultimately, a tremendous loss of somebody you cared a great deal about). To see yourself as damaged keeps you connected to her through a negative view of yourself. At times of stress the choice becomes unbearable."
>
> Through projective identification, this patient helped me to understand an important part of his inner experience. I was able to use the

material and play it back to him through a self-disclosure which he told me, weeks later, was the first time in his life he had felt fully understood.* The work continued as he came to understand how difficult it is to refute the picture of us held by those we love without feeling that the connection between that loved one and ourselves will be jeopardized. We thus look for ways, instead, of reconfirming that picture over and over in our interaction with others. Thus, a piece of mother's view, "You're bad and cause trouble," is carried around and reenacted as a way of confirming mother's view. The dilemma for the child (and the child within) is whether he can still love mother, and she him, if her view is wrong.

Another example occurred in a long-term group in which an alcoholic member had been "slipping." The week after her slip she came in and told the group leader, "I was mad that you didn't tell me I had to go to two AA meetings after my slip; but if you had, I wouldn't have done it because, as you know, it's important for me to be in control." To this, the therapist, aware of feeling stymied and frustrated, said, "I feel that I am doomed if I do and doomed if I don't, and in fact, that it's impossible to do anything right. I think this is a feeling that you know a good deal about and that lives in you much of the time."

My main objection to less-disciplined spontaneous self-disclosure is that it is often difficult to be clear about what is motivating the therapist. What the therapist feels is needed at the moment may be just what is needed, but I believe that it is useful to check out my impulses first before I do something unusual (and indeed, for many therapists, self-disclosure is relatively unusual).

Whether or not a particular self-disclosure is useful, it is also important to be aware that if self-disclosure is unusual for the therapist it will have impact that goes beyond the content of the particular self-disclosure. The fact that the leader has changed her role and modified the boundaries a bit can have an independent impact on the

---

*Such complicated and important interpretations often take weeks to be fully absorbed and digested, and are often met initially with confusion or other forms of resistance (adding to the importance of the therapist being crystal clear about what he is saying). For example, Mr. W interrupted me several times as I was making this interpretation, disputing my choice of one particular word or another. I had to deal with this resistance by interrupting the interpretation and wondering whether perhaps some part of him might be reluctant to hear what I was about to say. (Although being understood is something that we all yearn for, there may be considerable resistance against permitting this to happen—and against acknowledging it when it does.)

group, and the leader should be prepared to explore (or listen for) this. The following vignette illustrates the way in which a very small deviation from usual practice takes on great meaning, beyond the significance of the particular content of the self-disclosure.

> *Several months after I had removed my wedding ring, a patient with whom I had been working during the course of her own marital separation commented on my absent ring, and said very empathically, "I notice that your ring is gone and I don't know quite what it means, but I just hope that if you have been going through something difficult, there has been somebody there for you who has been as helpful and caring as you have been for me." Touched by her very personal comment, I suspect my eyes filled slightly, and I said simply, "Thank you." This was a small, brief response, but quite out of character—as it responded totally to the personal part of our relationship and her caring acknowledgment of me as a person. As brief as the intervention was the enormity of its impact. The patient immediately became distant—with a near paranoid accusation, "The trouble with psychotherapy is that it is such a cold, distant proposition. You never really know exactly what the therapist is thinking; it's all so one-sided!" She went on and on like this for about 2 minutes. When she stopped, I asked, "What just happened?" and she responded, "I guess for a moment there, we got too close." It should be noted that this response on my part was not one that was thought through, but was motivated by the fact that she had instantaneously touched me and I had spontaneously responded. I point to this example, not because I think that my behavior was so inappropriate, but because it illustrates how even small deviations are noticeable and important to pay attention to.*

Nonverbal Self-Disclosure of Feelings

Although, as the reader knows, I rarely directly state my feelings, it is clear from some of the examples in previous chapters that at times my feelings, particularly sadness, may show. Often I am asked how I make the decision to let this particular affect show (most often around termination). My decision about self-revelation in terms of letting my face express itself (although clearly this is not totally under my control) has to do with whether or not I believe the feeling that I will disclose is empathic and will be experienced as such by the patient. Sadness when a patient is terminating would generally be experienced empathically by the patient (unless the patient was not feeling sad). Anger, on the other hand, is more complicated. If I am angry at a patient's behavior or he is provoking me, it may not be at all empathic for me to communicate this anger (although I may use these feelings that are evoked in me to understand what may be going on in the group or in an individual member). On the other hand, if I am empathically outraged at the way another has treated my patient, my voice, expression, and demeanor might communicate this. For example, if a patient tells me blandly that someone has done something clearly outrageous to him, my tone might convey outrage if I felt that it would help the patient validate his own unexpressed rage. Thus, I might say, "He did what!" I might even say, "Are you serious?" The distinction I make in terms of whether I allow my feelings to become known to the patient hinges on whether I feel that my response is empathically attuned and will be perceived that way by the patient. In contrast, acting enraged when I am frustrated with a patient, would in most instances, I believe, give untherapeutic rein to my countertransference reactions—creating an unsafe atmosphere for the patient.

Thus, the decision about which of my feelings will show or will not show is not so much a matter of whether I am "honest" or not with all of my feelings, but rather, whether I think it is in the therapeutic interest of the patient to let the feelings be known. If a patient were talking about something sad and I found myself suddenly thinking about my own sadness, I would be more inclined to hold back. The gauge that I use to determine what and how much I will share is based on my assessment of the therapeutic utility for the patient—the extent to which I feel that my response is empathically attuned and will provide a mirror for the patient's feelings that will, ultimately, help him to be in touch with his own feelings. My empathic outrage is similarly used when it feels as if the response, not only is empathic, but will also help the patient get more in touch with his own appropriate rage.

Although, with regard to self-disclosure, I am at the conservative end of the spectrum and may even be viewed by some readers as "withholding"—a style that is often linked to extremely traditional psychoanalytic therapists, who are often seen as cold and unfriendly— the position that I take regarding self-disclosure, as I hope comes through in the style of my many interventions throughout the text, is not in any way related to being a cool, inactive therapist. On the contrary, particularly in my work as a group therapist, I am relatively active, use humor freely, and feel that a spirit of play on the leaders part is not inconsistent with the hard work that we expect of our patients (and ourselves).

LEADER SNAFUS

The Tongue-Tied Therapist: Making the Covert Overt

Often when a therapist feels tongue-tied or unable to communicate what she is feeling to a patient, it is because she fears that the communication will "leak" some feeling that she hopes to disguise. There is perfectly good language for most of the things that we want to say, except when we are trying desperately not to express part of it.

If the therapist has already been leaking it, making whatever it is overt is generally a relief to everyone—group members as well as the leader. In fact, the overt statement of the material is generally much easier to handle than the covert.

Let us take, for example, a group that has orchestrated an outside-of-group "social gathering" with all members present except the leader. The leader has felt reluctant about bringing this up and concerned about "leaking" the uncomfortable feelings that she has about this. It may be helpful for the leader to begin by asking herself what it is, exactly, that she is afraid to have the group know about her feelings? Perhaps this might be the leader's concern that she is not adequately meeting members' needs, or perhaps her own feelings of hurt and betrayal about their taking action without her. The group leader should ask herself two questions: First, do members already know what it is that she is trying to hide from them? (The answer is almost invariably, yes.) And second, if we discuss the issue overtly, what will be the consequences? Assuming that the material has already been leaked, making it overt should just make it more comfortable for everyone and provide relief to have it out in the open.

I am not suggesting here, as the reader might have guessed, given my general position on self-disclosure, that the leader share with the group that she has been feeling "hurt" or "betrayed," but rather, that she use these feelings as a signal of what the group may be wishing to communicate to her through their actions (and their intention to have an impact on the therapist). Thus, I might comment, "Perhaps group members have had a wish to keep me in the dark and feeling unaware of what was going on," or, "Perhaps there was a wish to have me feel a little left out—feelings that many of you have been experiencing in here."

Feeling Immobilized When the Group Needs to be Diverted

Often group leaders find themselves immobilized and unable to take action even when they have a clear sense that something is happening in the group that is getting in the way of group progress. Such leaders often feel that even relatively neutral questions to the group about how the group is doing, or whether the course they are on feels useful, will be taken as harsh criticism of the group. Often, leaders who experience this kind of conflict are, in fact, feeling extremely critical of the group and are afraid that any attempt to move the group (or a given patient) in a new direction will "leak out" the leader's disappointment. It may be helpful for the leader to consider that even good groups and good members often get sidetracked. Temporarily members may retreat, may filibuster, or may otherwise divert from a productive course. The leader needs to recognize that this happens in all groups. That the leader notices such diversions is not an indictment of the group (or the leader) but a recognition that the group needs help shifting in a slightly different direction.

Leader's Worst Fears: A Patient Will Be Extruded if the Leader Pulls for Direct Feedback

Often leaders are reluctant to help the group address a patient's dysfunctional (perhaps even obnoxious) behavior because the leader fears that members of the group do not really like that person (perhaps the leader doesn't either) and fears that if the group provides direct feedback, the person will be extruded from the group. Although it sometimes may happen that this kind of direct feedback will lead to the member's departure, it is important to be aware that this person would, in all likelihood, have departed even without the feedback. Group members, like all of us, are usually quite sensitive to other people's being disappointed, disgusted with them, or not liking them. If the feeling is in the room, it is likely that it has been perceived by the offending member, even if it is not being stated. In fact, it may even be contributing to increasing incidences of the obnoxious behavior. On the other hand, if the obnoxious behavior is addressed and the group talks about it openly and honestly, there is a chance that the offending member may come to understand her behavior better (and possibly modify it); and also that the group will come to understand her better and may become more tolerant. In my experience, little is lost by dealing directly with any problem, no matter how uncomfortable. If it is not dealt with, it never disappears spontaneously (even if the patient for some other "good reason" leaves the group).

The bottom line for all members in a group is that they have to come to feel that others in the group care about them. And if they are getting "vibes," no matter how subtle, that others don't care or don't understand, they are not going to continue in the group in any case. A caring discussion regarding the things about a member that others find objectionable allows an opportunity to talk about the behavior and, at the same time, to understand it. The behavior may not be liked, but the individual herself may still be accepted (and even loved).

It may also be possible for group members to understand that there is something about a given individual that "drives them nuts" because of something in their own past that it resonates with. Thus, a given member's obnoxious behavior may be obnoxious, not only by itself, but because it sets off particular kinds of reactions in other group members. This way of looking at the behavior suggests that part of what makes it difficult is interactional. Carol's behavior may drive the group crazy because she sets off something familiar and uncomfortable—possibly for one member because it is a characteristic in herself that she also hates, or for another member because "my mother used to torture me with that same kind of behavior." As the group starts talking about why a particular behavior is so hard for them, it becomes more empathically attuned to the offending member. To help with this, the leader might comment, "It sounds like you're saying, not only that Carol's style is hard, but also that it's especially hard for you because it's something in you that you have also tried hard to get rid of. What would it be like, do you think, if you and Carol were able to work on that together?" Or, to the person who says that he doesn't like Carol, the leader might comment, "It sounds like there's a real opportunity here to learn something about yourself and how you manage these kinds of situations."

Difficult group situations pose an opportunity for learning and for growth. Thus, I might say, "My hunch is that there is a real opportunity in this for us to understand better what's going on and what's pushing a lot of people's buttons, even though it does feel pretty painful right now." Or the leader might say to the group, "This is a very tough place to be right now, but my hunch is that as we come to understand it better, it will provide a real opportunity for everyone in here. Even though feelings are strong right now, or perhaps *because* the feelings are so strong, there is a real chance to grow if we're not afraid of it."

Leader Fears a Topic May Be Too Hot for the Group: The Possibility of a Need for Additional Therapy

Often during the course of a long-term therapy group, an issue comes up that is especially loaded for a particular patient—raising the question of need for other therapeutic support in addition to the group. For example, an incest victim may bring up, for the first time, her history of sexual abuse—displaying considerable affect and pain. The initial reaction of group leaders (and/or members) may reflect their own discomfort with the material and the feeling that the issue would be better dealt with somewhere else. Or the patient herself may suggest that she should deal with it elsewhere—fearing that she may overwhelm the group. Sometimes, in such situations it may be useful for the patient to have additional therapeutic support—perhaps the addition of an individual therapist, or even an additional group, particularly if it is time limited and focuses on the crisis issue (e.g., an incest group). On the other hand, I think it is important that group leaders and the group (as well as the member who brings up the emotionally loaded material) consider carefully what is motivating the quest for additional support. Although in many instances this request may be quite reasonable, the message regarding the need for additional support should not imply that the topic is "too hot" for the group or something that "can't be talked about here." I do not believe that there is any topic that "does not belong" in a therapy group. All topics are appropriate as long as patients are given the help they need in processing and adequately containing their feelings.

Countertransference Leakage in Letters Sent to Patients

The patient who mysteriously disappears from the group and cannot be reached by phone creates complicated communication challenges for the group leader. It is generally useful, under such circumstances, to write a letter indicating that it is important that the group member be in touch and that he let the group know where he stands in terms of his membership. It may also be useful in such a letter to remind the patient of his agreement, prior to joining the group, that he would discuss with the group any thoughts about leaving (if that is, indeed, his intention). The letter should be encouraging and inviting—an attempt to reengage the member. But it is also important that the letter communicate a clear time frame for getting back to the leaders, with a message that if he has not been in touch by a specified date, they will assume that he is not currently interested in pursuing his relationship with the group and that they will let the group know that he is no longer a member.

In addition to clarifying the patient's status with regard to the group, the tone and content of the letter are important in terms of the patient's future therapeutic work—in terms of resuming treatment either with you or with another treater in the future. Often by the time group leaders get to the point of writing such letters they are already feeling, understandably, quite frustrated by the wavering patient and the time they have already spent trying to reach him, unsuccessfully, by phone. Also, they may be feeling abandoned and rejected by the patient and perhaps even humiliated that they have not been able to provide a more definitive statement for the rest of the group. All these are very natural and understandable feelings. Generally speaking, however, it is not in the best interest of the patient (the recipient of such a letter) for these feelings to be "leaked." If, as is generally our hope, we want the patient to return to treatment (if not at this point, at least at some future point), it is important that the letter have a genuinely inviting and open tone. Often leaders intend this to be so, but their anger, disappointment, and frustration "leak" through in the tone of the letter. (Dead giveaways are business language and phraseology—words such as "wherein," "hence," "in light of," "whereupon." Sprinklings of colons and semicolons may also serve as red lights.)

To avoid countertransference leakage, it is a good idea to ask somebody else who is not intimately connected to the situation (your co-therapist, who is also frustrated and disappointed, is not a very helpful candidate for this) to read the letter. Ask this person simply, "If you got this letter, how would you feel?" And also, "If you got this letter, would you want to come back to our group or to other therapy in the future?" In fact, it is probably the case that almost any letter written to a patient would benefit by a review from a colleague—since almost anytime you find it necessary to write, it is because the usual forms of communication have already been blocked in some way.

The Leader Who Worries about Patient Catharsis and Specific Agendas

Sometimes group leaders worry excessively about patients who participate around other group members' material and seem actively engaged but do not specifically bring up material of their own. However, it is important for leaders to remember that group members gain from a therapy group in many different ways. Chief among these is the feeling of connectedness to other group members as well as the opportunity to learn more about "how people tick." Much of this learning (what people are about and how they connect to one another) can take place even during periods when a given member is disclosing relatively little in terms of personal material about herself. It is likely, as she engages with others, that the things she chooses to latch on to are meaningful to herself as well, and that through this route, she is also coming to do an important part of the task that she is there for.

Sometimes group leaders have the feeling that, without tremendous catharsis on the part of each group member, no group growth will take place. I do not believe that "purging one's guts" is essential. In fact, we often find that patients who come in session after session and "purge" (either in individual or group therapy), exhaust both themselves and the therapist (as well as other group members) to such an extent that there is little energy left over to process the mess. Coming in and "throwing up" week after week may even be used defensively to avoid exploring what is going on inside. To put it differently, the purpose of group psychotherapy (or any psychotherapy) is not to spill out the contents of one's gut but to *understand* what is in there.

A related problem for group leaders is that they sometimes come to believe that there is some *specific* thing that a patient has to talk about in the group. They worry when the patient is not talking enough about "it", or become concerned when they have not heard about "it" in a while. However, the notion that the work of therapy has to do with discussing some *particular thing* misses the point of a therapy group. What is important is that members come to understand that they *can* talk about all aspects of themselves—that there is nothing so reprehensible that it must be hidden—and that they can remain feeling connected to people and accepted, even when they do share this personal information. This does not mean that the material has to be shared repeatedly. As a leader I am less concerned about whether the patient talks about some particular item than about whether the patient feels connected to the group. With the exception of pressing life crises (including relapses and "near misses"), it is helpful if leaders can free themselves from the feeling that there is a particular topic or agenda from the past that a patient must deal with in order to do the work of the group.

It is also important to note that, for new members in particular, sharing of certain kinds of personal information too soon can actually be used defensively. For example, a new member in the first session or two may "spill her guts" about some highly personal and charged material that, in fact, pushes the group away and makes her feel alienated and separate (she shared too much too soon). When we consider the real energy of the group, it is generally in the here and now—what people share in the present with one another and come to learn about themselves in the arena of the group. In a sense, the outside-of-group material just provides a handle for that task. As most group leaders are aware, the group is liveliest when there are interactions going on between people in the present. The narratives about the past or about current relationships outside the group are only as lively as the current connections that they induce within the group.

Leader Absences

Group leaders often have complicated feelings about their own absences from the group and how best to care for the group when they must be away. Some leaders handle their "vacations" and other absences from the group by canceling the group, others allow their groups to meet without them, and still others provide a covering therapist (Rutan, Alonso, & Molin, 1984).* I prefer the latter because it not only provides greater continuity than not meeting and greater safety than allowing the group to meet alone but, in addition, it introduces important thematic material from the past. All of us had parents who were away at some point and experienced alternate coverage with a baby sitter. Thus, this model introduces many of the important feelings and dynamics from that old familiar situation— including splitting. This can take the form of either the baby sitter being seen as the good parent and the absent therapist as the bad one who has abandoned them —or, conversely, the absent therapist may be seen as the good one (despite her abandoning ways), and the baby sitter may get the flak. It is important to recognize that the feelings that come up toward the substitute leader (as well as the regular leader) need to be explored and not just taken at face value and, also, need to be reintegrated into the group.

When one group told the leader upon her return how "wonderful" the substitute was and how much fun they had when the leader was away, the message was clearly "who needs you anyway—it's a lot more fun when you're gone." In another group, when the leader left for 2 months to have a baby, all the rage that the patients felt toward the departing leader got focused on the "withholding" substitute. Upon her return, the leader had to help the group understand the rage they felt toward her for her own substantial withholding (depriving them of herself altogether) for a period of some 8 weeks. In yet another group, the leader upon her return from a 2-week absence, was greeted by a proclamation from one group member, "I hate gray-haired mothers with strollers"—thinly veiled rage at the gray-haired leader who had "strolled" from the group.

In my experience, if patients know in advance that whenever the leader is away there will be alternate coverage and this is an accepted part of how the group operates, business in the group goes on "as usual" (or almost) with the substitute leader. Substitute coverage also provides a wonderful learning vehicle for the therapist who goes away—an opportunity to see her group through the eyes of a new

---

*These alternatives all assume that there is not a co-leader who will be present.

viewer. Groups (as a way of "getting even" with the absent leader) may also disclose previously undisclosed material that is bound to be useful to the group in its ongoing work. The group should be encouraged to talk with the leader when she returns about what it was like when she was gone, and it should be clear that she and the covering leader will talk (both before the absence and after). There should be no sense in the group that what happened with the covering therapist is separate and apart from the usual group—but rather, that whatever came up is relevant to the ongoing work of the group.

Finally, substitute coverage provides a wonderful opportunity for the covering therapist, who has a chance to sample, first hand, a group other than her own. In a clinic setting such as ours, where group placement decisions are made with collective input from a clinic team, this provides the additional advantage of having many people who are familiar with each of the groups and facilitates placement of patients in groups where they will be a good fit.

CO-LEADERSHIP

Benefits and Costs

Co-leadership offers a number of special benefits both to the group leaders and to the group members. Leaders gain from the opportunity to have peer support during the group itself and to have easy access to backup coverage for holidays and vacations. In addition, the prospect of sharing the rich and fascinating experience of group life makes it even more fun. Leaders also benefit, in terms of their own growth as therapists, by having an opportunity to watch another therapist work. The sharing of responsibility and the decreased sense of burden that often accompanies this, as well as the ability to give constructive feedback to one another, help leaders to stay on top of the intricate, and sometimes confusing, dynamics of the group.

From the perspective of group members, benefits include the opportunity to watch functional, adaptive behavior in the co-leader pair—a real bonus for many patients from dysfunctional families, who have had little opportunity to observe open dyadic communication and sharing of adult responsibility. In addition, particularly with a male/female co-therapy team, co-leadership enhances the "re-creation of the family" and the group's capacity to fully play out the many dimensions of family transference. Co-leadership for many patients may also diffuse the transference (particularly feelings around dependency and loss), since there is not just a single "parent" to rely on. Finally, co-leadership provides an opportunity for two sets of eyes to view the situation, rather than one, and for the patients to benefit from the leaders' collaboration.

Along with the many benefits of co-leadership, however, there are also some important costs that need to be considered.* In private practice, co-leadership is generally less financially rewarding for the therapist. (In clinics, co-leadership generally also adds to the clinic costs—unless the co-therapist is an unpaid trainee.) In addition, the co-leaders need to allow extra time after each group session to process the group material with one another and to discuss future interventions and clinical strategies. Finally, co-therapy adds an additional leader responsibility, since the leaders must take the time to attend to their own relationship. Leaders must be prepared to talk about what is going on between them, to explore differences, to deal with sexual attractions to one another without acting on them, and to be open to understanding how issues that come up between them may be reflected in the work of the group. The importance of this cannot be underestimated. Group members will be sensitive to tensions between the leaders, just as children are ever sensitive to tensions between their parents. Even when the group does not directly address these issues, they inadvertently get played out in the group, and if the leaders are discerning, they will ultimately hear the material and be able to process it with the group.

A common initial issue among co-therapists has to do with competition and division of functions within the group. Often co-leaders worry that they may be talking too much or too little relative to the other partner—or have concerns about whether they need to pull back to offset the other who is more active or, alternatively, to give the other a chance. Similarly, at times one therapist has one thing in mind in terms of the direction that he is hoping the group will move clinically, and the other makes a move that goes in the opposite direction. Leaders need to be tolerant of their differences but also need to work

---

*See Dick, Lessler, and Whiteside (1980) and Dies (1983) for reviews of the literature on advantages and disadvantages of co-therapy.

out ways of combining their efforts so that a move by one leader in one direction does not necessarily close the door to a different move by the other. For example, leaders may work out a style in which they can validate the direction in which one leader was moving and add to it by saying, "In addition to the point that Jim (the other co-therapist) was making, it also occurred to me that . . . ."

Issues of competition may also come up as each leader worries whether group members like him as much as they like the other leader, respect him as much, use his interpretations as much, or are as likely to bring material back into the group that he has raised. These kinds of "comparisons" are an underestimated part of sharing a project in which both parties want very much to feel competent and in control. Like any close, successfully interactive relationship, the co-therapy relationship must be constantly attended to, and constant recalibration is necessary. In this regard the similarities between co-therapy and marriage have been noted by several authors (Heilfron, 1969; Dick et al., 1980), highlighting the importance of open communication as well as each partner's awareness and acceptance of his own and his partner's talents and limitations.

Choosing a Co-Leader

In choosing a co-leader a balance must be struck between comfortable similarities and profitable differences between the two leaders. Although many combinations are possible and workable, differences between the leaders (as long as they are within a comfortable range) can provide richness for the group. For this reason, I prefer male-female combinations whenever possible, and personal and stylistic differences within a range that the leaders can comfortably tolerate. Probably the most important criteria are that the leaders generally like and respect one another, look forward to working together, and anticipate that their work will be both fun and rewarding.

If after meeting a potential co-leader you have any reservations about your comfort in working together, this should be discussed at length, prior to making a commitment to co-leadership. Counterindications for a co-therapy pair include the following: (1) differences in clinical orientation which the leaders believe will be conflictual (for example, one leader who is very traditionally trained and analytically oriented, and another whose training is in transactional analysis or

Gestalt therapy); (2) tremendous disparity in activity level, which the leaders may already know about from their contacts with one another outside the group (for example, one leader is extremely active, emotional, and affectively available, and the other is extremely reserved and finds high activity and emotionality irksome); (3) negative attraction between the two group leaders (for example, when two group leaders find themselves disliking one another or when one finds the other unappealing personally); (4) uncomfortable positive attraction (for example, when one or both of the leaders have had thoughts of dating the other or of having an affair—unless they can comfortably give up acting on these wishes); and (5) a negative history together that one or both leaders cannot get past.

Many group therapists believe that co-leadership also requires that the leaders are nearly coequal in status. However, in my own experience, supervising more than 200 co-leader pairs over the last 17 years,* I believe that status "equality" is nearly impossible to achieve, and that a considerable amount of inequality can be managed as long as the leaders are aware of the differences (and the implications for their work together) and are receptive to processing this as "grist for the mill" in the group and in supervision. Considering the many possible status differentials among people, it is hard to imagine a truly coequal pair (and certainly not "coequal" in the eyes of all group members, since each will have his own yardstick to use for measuring equality). The perceived status of various professional disciplines differ; age carries with it differential status since it is often associated with different amounts of experience; experience levels may vary independently of age (and also independent of number of years of actual work in the field); gender may carry differential status for some members (and for some leaders); and so on.

In addition, particularly in long-term groups that go on for years and in which there is co-leader turnover, the newer leader will almost always be perceived as having a lower status than the one who has been there longer. In my experience, nearly every group has a big "C" (the more senior co-leader) and a little "C" (the less senior co-leader). In our clinic, in fact, such an arrangement helps provide training for

---

*Some 75 of these pairs were together for a year or more in long-term groups; another 125 in short-term (5-week) groups.

group leaders beginning their work in this field. What is important is that the status differentials between the leaders are not uncomfortable for them, that they can listen for issues related to these differences and deal with them appropriately when they come up in the group, and that the leaders make every effort to divide the work load of the group as evenly as possible. Despite status differentials (actual or perceived), the work load can and should be shared, and impediments to this (for example, the senior leader having difficulty sharing his group with a new co-leader) should be discussed.

Co-Leadership Variations When the Co-Leader Is a Trainee

In many institutions where group psychotherapy is conducted, neo-phyte therapists "learn the trade" by an apprenticeship model in which they pair up with more senior group psychotherapists. This is a work-able model as long as both the more senior co-therapist (the big C) and the more junior co-therapist (the little C) are aware of the discrep-ancies and are willing to tolerate that one is likely to be seen as more senior than the other and that the less experienced leader is willing to, in a sense, learn and take the lead from the big C. In my experience, the group can tolerate a fair amount of disparity between the skills of the two co-therapists as long as the two therapists themselves are relatively comfortable with this and have discussed it, and as long as it is open for comment and discussion in the group as well. For this model to work, however, it is also essential that the little C have some clinical skills (i.e., is not totally green to the therapeutic culture and has an understanding of the ways in which group therapy works).

If the disparity between the co-leaders is very great (because of the relatively unsophisticated clinical skills of the trainee), an alternative model may be to use the trainee as a "recorder" in the group. This gives the trainee an opportunity to sit in a live group, week after week observing the process, with an opportunity for dialogue with the group leader afterwards and to participate in an ongoing supervision. The recorder may also take process notes, either during or immedi-ately after the group. I prefer to have the recorder take notes during the group because it gives her something to do while in the group and makes it easier to remain relatively opaque and nontransparent. It also makes overt and real what the group will be told about her presence in the room. In our clinic we tell groups, "From time to time, groups have a recorder along with the therapist in order to help keep track of what is going on in the group. The role of the recorder in here will be to help me keep track of what's happening so that when I think about it afterwards, I will have more of a handle on it." Some group leaders prefer to have the recorder sit in the circle with the rest of the group, others right outside the group circle; I have had experience with both and find them both workable.

Alternatively, a less experienced co-therapist can be given a more circumscribed role in the group with a repertoire of "safe" responses that will keep him involved and a "presence" in the group without interfering with the group movement that is being facilitated by the more senior therapist. Thus, the little C may be given the task of opening and closing the group, making initial announcements, underscoring interventions made by the big C, and asking for clarifications and further elaborations. The little C can mirror responses of the big C that need to be underscored. For example, the big C has just asked a patient what his reaction was to another member's comment. If this question goes unanswered, the little C a few minutes later might say, "A few minutes ago, Bob (big C) asked you how you were feeling about Carol's response to you, and I wonder what reaction you had to Bob's question." Thus, the little C can ask about people's reactions to interventions that the big C has made which go unexamined, or he can simply restate the same intervention—both relatively easy tasks to take on (basically forwarding a motion that has already begun). The little C can also ask for more information, "Can you say a little more about that?" or "How do you mean?" That is, very light exploratory questions that simply get him into the process and help move it in a positive direction.

Other more sophisticated kinds of interventions—interpretations, moving the group from one place to another, disagreements with the co-therapist, etc., should be noted (to herself) by the little C during the group and discussed afterwards. As time goes by and the little C has an opportunity to validate the useful things that she would have said and gains understanding of some of the maneuvers and strategies used by the more senior therapist, she will become increasingly able to take on these interventions herself.

It should be noted that the function of co-therapists is often not only to provide training for the junior co-therapist but to provide support for the big C. And even a recorder may be useful for this, since there is another observer to help keep track of what is going on and to help provide a clear perspective when the group is over.

Processing and Understanding Co-Therapy Conflicts

Our understanding of countertransference dynamics—and, in particular, the ways in which the therapist becomes a "container" (Bion, 1962) for important, conflictual feelings in the group—can be applied to the co-therapy team as a unit. Thus, when conflicts emerge between the two group leaders, it may be fruitful to examine the possibility that the co-therapist unit is experiencing two sides of a conflict—with one part being experienced by one therapist, and the other part by the other. (That is, the group is "impressing" one part of the conflict on one member of the co-therapy team, and another part on the other.) As discussed earlier in this chapter, in the course of therapy certain of the patients' unacceptable feelings may get projected out and "contained" by the group leader, whose resonance with the material and ability to understand what he is experiencing make it possible for him to "digest it" and put it back out for the group, or individual group members, to use. This occurs in a similar fashion within the co-leader dyad. Whereas with one leader, the patient (or group) puts out a part of the conflict so that it will be externalized (and experienced as a struggle with the leader), with two leaders, the group (or given patient) has an opportunity to externalize both parts of the conflict—leaving the leaders to represent the polarities, and to "fight it out between themselves" (with the group members freed up to "observe the conflict").

It is essential that the leaders in this situation use their understanding of the conflict between themselves as a way to better understand the feuding, intrapsychic positions within the group (and within individual members). These moments of tension, when the leaders experience conflict between themselves, can be important turning points if the leaders use their understanding of the conflict between themselves as a way of better gauging what is going on in the group. Of course, the reverse is also true: when tension remains within the co-leader team, it interferes with the progress of the group, often serving as a major distraction (for group members, as well as for the leaders). It is one of the greatest challenges of co-leadership to be able to understand and use the dyadic conflicts that emerge. Good supervision, or at least consultation with a respected colleague, is essential during these periods of conflict.

This chapter has discussed therapist's roadblocks including countertransference issues and confusion about the therapeutic stance. In addition, the costs and benefits of co-therapy were addressed along with the role of co-therapy in training. The next chapter deals with the training and preparation that are essential for the therapist if he is to competently oversee the group's journey.

❖ 11 ❖
Group Leader Preparation and Training

with DALE DILLAVOU, Ph.D.

It is important for the group therapist working in the field of substance abuse to be knowledgeable about substance abuse and how it affects those who are themselves chemically dependent, as well as the significant others who interact with them. In addition, training and preparation in group psychotherapy are essential. This chapter outlines the content areas necessary for the training and preparation of the group therapist working in the field of substance abuse, readings that will be helpful, and specialized group therapy training experiences that are available.

Information about Substance Abuse

Knowledge about substance abuse is important for initial clinical assessment and appropriate triage, not only for treating the substance abuser but for treating family members as well, since (as described in Chapter 3) many ACOAs and other significant others who present for treatment may themselves have problems with substance abuse or may be worried about it. In addition, knowledge will reduce the likelihood of countertransference alliances around myths, misbeliefs, and negative stereotypes about alcohol and drug abusers. The latter is important because many therapists who are drawn to working in the field of substance abuse will have had some personal or familial experience with substance abuse. These personal experiences, while creating a sense of familiarity with some of the issues, do not constitute adequate knowledge. Ironically, therapists who see themselves as having "lived through" some aspect of substance abuse (either in their own personal histories or in that of a loved one) may be especially vulnerable to stereotyped views and negative countertransference reactions to substance abusers, which may impede the therapist's ability to work effectively and to help group members clarify some of their own faulty thinking. Thus, the therapist working with substance abusers and their families and close associates will benefit from knowing more about substance abuse—the many courses it may take and the many ways it may become entwined in the family system.

Complexity of the Problem and Heterogeneity among Substance Abusers

Because substance abuse is a complex, multifaceted problem, the therapist working in this field needs to be sensitive to the physiological, medical, psychological, behavioral, and interpersonal consequences of substance abuse and the interplay among these consequences. Substance abuse affects many different kinds of people and in different ways. This tremendous diversity, even within the alcohol field alone, has given rise to a current view among alcololologists that it is more correct to refer to the "alcoholisms" rather than to alcoholism (Zucker, 1987)—a change in terminology meant to capture the considerable variety among people who become alcoholics (Pattison, 1985), the symptoms that they manifest (Cloninger, 1987; Pattison, 1985), the course of the illness (Cahalan, 1976; Clark & Cahalan, 1976), the course of recovery (Polich, Armor, & Braiker, 1981), and the treatment options that are the most effective. There are few simple "generalizable facts" that are true of all alcoholics (despite the presence of a myriad of unsubstantiated but dearly held beliefs about alcoholism that pervade both the alcoholic and nonalcoholic communities). The same can be said about substance abuse more generally. Understanding the severity of an alcohol or drug problem requires more than simply knowing the frequency or quantity of usage, when and how it is used, or the physiological or psychological sequelae. What appears to be "alcoholism" or "drug abuse" under one cultural microscope may look different in a population with a different age group or different cultural background. It is also important to know whether the patient is abusing more than one chemical substance (as is more and more frequently the case) and how these various substances interact. For the dual-diagnosis patient on antipsychotic and antidepressant medications, the patient's "balancing act" between what his doctor prescribes and his own self-medication must also be attended to. Each of these factors is important and must be considered, but only in combination do we understand the full picture. The therapist must be trained to attend to the heterogeneity among substance abusers.

Because substance abuse is so complex and requires more than "common- sense" understanding, we encourage the reader to expand his knowledge about it (and have provided an annotated bibliography to assist in selecting readings). Our hope is that the reader will develop a sense that much of what he already "knows" may not be entirely accurate. On a more optimistic note, the "truths" that we would pass on are the following: (1) People do not set out to become chemically dependent. Substance abuse arises out of a complex interplay of predisposing genetic factors, psychological factors, and sociocultural factors (Shaffer & Gambino, 1990). We are far from totally understanding the complex interplay. (2) Many substance abusers do get better (Saxe, Dougherty, Esty, & Fine, 1983; Vaillant et al., 1983; Washton, 1989; Washton, Gold, & Pottash, 1986), and when they do the quality of their lives and those of their families is often indistinguishable from that of individuals who were not formerly chemically dependent (Moos & Billings, 1982; Moos, Finney, & Chan, 1981; Moos & Moos, 1984; Vaillant, 1983). (3) Finally, treatment is available.

Treatment for Substance Abuse

Understanding when treatment is needed and the important components of treatment is clearly essential for effective clinical intervention. Most experts in the field of substance abuse agree that treatment begins with bringing the substance-abuse problem under control, though there may be some disagreement about whether this means behavioral control and management of the use (Pattison, 1985; Polich, Armor, & Braiker, 1980; Sobell & Sobell, 1973a, 1973b, 1976; Marlatt, 1985) or total abstinence (Vaillant et al., 1983; Washton, 1989; Weisman & Robe, 1983; Zimberg, 1982). Treatment is generally thought to be indicated when substance use has significant negative consequences in any area of the patient's life (physical or psychological health, relationships, employment), yet the use of substances persists (Pattison, 1985). Increasingly, clinicians who treat the problem recognize that by the time treatment is indicated, (1) the substance abuse has developed a life and a momentum of its own which needs to be treated in its own right (that is, the alcohol or drug problem will not go away by itself simply because the underlying, or accompanying, problems are being treated); and (2) halting the substance abuse makes it possible for the patient to deal more effectively with other problems that may exist. For these and other reasons, often the most crucial decision that the clinician will make is to address the substance abuse first, directly, and firmly (Khantzian, 1985; Levin, 1987; Steinglass et al, 1987; Vannicelli, 1982; Vannicelli et al., 1988; Washton, 1989; Zimberg, 1982).

Treatment options today are extensive and include a wide array of inpatient and outpatient programs of varying length and intensity. Although clinical research has not documented the superiority of the more costly and restrictive inpatient option over the less costly and more flexible alternative of outpatient treatment (Miller & Hester, 1986; Saxe et al., 1983), clinical judgment often points to inpatient treatment when withdrawal becomes complicated or when outpatient treatment has not proven effective. In our experience we have found that outpatient treatment is often extremely effective in supporting and facilitating the long-term work of recovery (Vannicelli, 1978) and that group psychotherapy, in particular, offers many advantages (Griefen, Vannicelli, & Canning, 1985; Vannicelli, 1982, 1987, 1988; Vannicelli et al., 1984, 1988). We also believe that AA and NA are highly synergistic with good professional treatment, and that patients should be encouraged to use these self-help programs. Patients' initial resistance can often be addressed by examining obstacles to participation. Individual, family, and couples therapy are also often extremely helpful. Finally, disulfiram (Antabuse) treatment can also be a very useful adjunct to assist in impulse control during the early stages of recovery. (See the Annotated Bibliography at the end of this chapter for a guide to reading about alcoholism and substance abuse.)

Information about the Family

Understanding what it means to be a member of an "alcoholic family" is obviously at the heart of our work with ACOAs and collaterals. But it is important to be familiar with the considerable diversity that exists among alcoholic families. Until recently the accepted view of alcoholism and the alcoholic family had been based largely on the relatively few alcoholics who found their way into treatment. By broadening our knowledge base and by understanding the ways in which alcohol may be used in the family systems of those who never reach treatment for their alcoholism, we broaden our sense of what our ACOA patients may have experienced.

The work of Steinglass and his colleagues (Steinglass et al., 1987; Wolin, Bennett, & Noonan, 1979) documents the ways in which alcohol is used by the entire family system and the ways in which it may (or may not) be entwined in the life and rituals of the family. This work also helps us to understand intergenerational transmission and identity issues around alcoholism, as well as the centrality (or lack thereof) of the "ACOA" identity.

Group Psychotherapy Preparation

The group therapist undertaking this enterprise should have solid training and supervision in group psychotherapy. As Dies (1983) and Friedman (1989) point out, skill in individual therapy does not automatically "transfer" to the group-therapy setting. Moreover, experience alone does not develop skill, as demonstrated by a study (Ebersole, Leiderman, & Yalom, 1969) of 13 beginning group therapists, 7 of whom participated in an experimental condition in which training and supervision were provided, and 6 of whom participated in a control condition in which no supervision and training were provided. Observer ratings by trained clinicians 6 months later indicated that while the performance of the therapists who had received training improved, performance of those assigned to the control group actually deteriorated. These authors conclude that unsupervised experience may result in reinforcement of original errors and misconceptions.

Friedman (1989) addresses this issue further by pointing out that, although most licenses permit the professional to do anything that anyone in his profession is competent to do (e.g., a psychiatrist can legally do surgery under his medical license), codes of ethics prohibit the delivery of services if one lacks adequate preparation. Thus, as he puts it, "It is certainly unethical for a fully credentialed professional to begin on-the-job training in group therapy without competent, on-going supervision in *that* modality" (p. 19, italics added).

Formal training in group psychotherapy may be accomplished via a number of routes. Clinical psychology graduate programs, schools of social work, and many allied disciplines offer course work in group psychotherapy. In addition, the local divisions of the American Group Psychotherapy Association (both state and regional) offer 1-, 2-, and 3-year training programs in group psychotherapy. Excellent textbooks on outpatient group psychotherapy include those authored by Yalom (1975), Vinogradov and Yalom (1989) (a concise paperback), Corey and Corey (1987), and Rutan and Stone (1984).

Finally, hands-on supervised experience is essential. We do not recommend that even an experienced therapist begin her first substance-abuse group or group for collaterals totally on her own. The level of supervision or supervisory consultation will depend on the general level of clinical expertise of the therapist and, in particular, the amount of prior experience doing group psychotherapy. Experienced therapists who are knowledgeable about group psychotherapy with other populations may wish to simply begin this enterprise with peer supervision (i.e., collaborating with other colleagues who are also doing a substance-abuse group or a group for collaterals of substance abusers). Collaboration with an experienced co-therapist may be sufficient if a provision is made for back-up consultation for the occasional impasses that may develop. Therapists embarking on this venture with less group-psychotherapy experience are advised to have regular supervision (weekly or biweekly), either individually or in a supervision group. While individual supervision provides greater opportunity for regular and continuous monitoring of the therapist's own particular group, the supervision group provides an opportunity to learn by listening to the snafus and glitches encountered in other groups (as well as their resolution). The former format may be less anxiety provoking initially, particularly when the therapist feels somewhat pressed about staying on top of the process in her own group (and anxious about the prospect of many observers witnessing the rough spots encountered along the way). As competence grows, however, the group supervision format has much to recommend it, since "parallel process" often develops in the supervision group, paralleling the issues and conflicts in members' own individual groups and providing a particularly rich arena for exploring countertransference phenomena.

If group supervision is used—with or without a leader—we prefer a format that deviates slightly from the usual approach, which tends to begin (at least the first time the group is presented) with a lengthy review of the cast of characters, their histories, and presenting problems. Though this approach has a certain inherent logic, it is generally very difficult for other peer group members to keep track of the cast of characters until they have something more meaty on which to hang the character descriptions. Sometimes it is even hard to stay tuned in. The format that we prefer is to omit the particulars of each member until they are relevant to answering meaningful questions about what is going on in the group. We often find it helpful to begin with the following questions, which are equally useful if a single session is being presented, or if the presentation is following the format of the group "up till now."

1. What is the group as a whole working on (themes and issues)?
2. How well are they doing at it? (What are the blocks or resistances, and what positive forces exist in the group to help the group move ahead?)
3. How do members relate to one another in the group (as well as outside, if this is relevant)?
4. How do the leaders feel about the work that the group is doing?

Readings in the Field of Substance Abuse

We have provided an annotated bibliography of substance-abuse readings in three categories—readings about substance abuse, readings about adult children of alcoholics, and readings about work with other collaterals of substance abusers (spouses and other family members). These are important, informative readings that will add considerably to the depth and breadth of the therapist's understanding of the substance-abuse field, including research relevant to many of the clinical conceptualizations outlined in this book.

In addition to the informative papers in our annotated bibliography, there is an enormous lay literature in the substance-abuse field, including many self-help books. Many patients, particularly those who present for treatment as ACOAs, have sampled from the vast self-help literature available, and the therapist may want to be familiar with some of these as well (Ackerman, 1986, 1987; Birke & Mayer, 1990; Black, 1981, 1985; Cermak, 1985; Friel & Friel, 1988; Gravitz & Bowden, 1985; Greenleaf, 1981; Kritsberg, 1985; McConnell, 1980, 1986; McDonnell & Callahan, 1987; Middleton-Moz & Dwinell,

1986; Miller & Ripper, 1988; Seixas & Youcha, 1985; Smith, 1988; Wegscheider-Cruse, 1985; Whitfield, 1987; Woititz, 1983, 1985). ACOAs often find these books extremely helpful; they feel personally connected to and identify with the ideas, and in many instances these readings have also been instrumental in getting them into treatment. That the ideas expressed in these lay books are broad enough that many non-ACOA patients (and probably most of their therapists as well) will also identify with them, in no way lessens the impact on a particular ACOA client who finds these readings useful. These books are intended for the lay public and for that audience have considerable appeal. However, they should be read with a grain of salt by the therapist looking for "factual information" about ACOAs, since overgeneralizations and somewhat stereotyped characterizations are pervasive in this literature. Since the content of these books overlaps considerably, it probably makes most sense to choose whichever books are most available or those which your clients seem to be talking about the most.

An equally large array of self-help books is available for other collaterals (Drews, 1980; Forrest, 1986; Johnson, 1986; Becnel, 1989; Beattie, 1987, 1990a, 1990b; Alexander & Alexander, 1991; Mellody & Miller, 1989; Porterfield, 1984; Schlesinger & Horberg, 1988; Subby, 1990), as well as for the substance abuser himself (Carnes, 1989; Secil, 1990; Mueller & Ketcham 1987; Mummey, 1987; Nuckols, 1989; O'Connel, 1985; Paine-Gernee & Hunt, 1990; Pittman, 1988; Smith, 1990). Although patients may also find many of these helpful, the caution advised above regarding the lay ACOA literature is equally applicable to much of this literature.

Annotated Bibliography of Readings

Substance Abusers

American Psychiatric Association. *Diagnostic and statistical manual of mental disorders (3rd ed., Rev.).* Washington, DC: American Psychiatric Association, 1987. (pp. 116-185)

> These sections of DSM-III-R contain very useful descriptive information. Intoxication and withdrawal are detailed for alcohol, cocaine, marijuana, barbiturates, PCP, and other drugs. Other drug-related states such as alcohol hallucinocis, cocaine delirium, and cannabis delusional disorder are defined. The sections providing diagnostic criteria for the various

psychoactive substance-use disorders reflect an increased recognition of the importance of psychosocial factors in determining dependence. A very useful reference.

Blane, H.T., and Leonard, K.E. (Eds). *Psychological theories of drinking and alcoholism.* New York: Guilford, 1987.

An authoritative account of current theory and programmatic research regarding alcoholism. This book provides a stimulating array of points of view. Each chapter presents a theoretical conceptualization, research findings that bear upon it, and an assessment of its strengths and weaknesses. This is an important book for a field that is too often stifled by adherence to unchallenged beliefs.

Brownell, K.D., Marlatt, G.A, Lichtenstein, E., and Wilson, G.T. Understanding and preventing relapse. *American Psychologist,* 1986, *41,* 765-782.

Written by cognitive behaviorists, this article looks at relapse from a psychological rather than biomedical point of view. Knowledge gained from the study of several kinds of addictive disorders (alcoholism, smoking, and obesity) is examined for commonalities.

Clark, W., and Cahalan, D. Changes in drinking over a four-year span. *Addictive Behaviors,* 1976, *1,* 251-259.

Longitudinal study of drinking problems documenting the variability in the nature of drinking problems and in their course.

Cook, D.R. Craftsman versus professional: Analysis of the controlled drinking controversy. *Journal of Studies on Alcohol,* 1985, *46,* 433-442.

An attempt to understand and depolarize the controversy centered on the Sobells' controlled drinking study and criticism of their conclusions by Pendry et al. (*Science,* 1985, *217,* 169-175).

Donovan, D.M., and Marlatt, G.A. Assessment of expectancies and behaviors associated with alcohol consumption. *Journal of Studies on Alcohol,* 1980, *41,* 1153-1185.

The authors take a systematic look at the research data bearing on many of the old saws and myths in the field of alcoholism—in particular regarding tension-reduction theories of alcoholism, loss of control, craving, and mood changes and other psychological conditions during the course of alcoholism.

Donovan, D. and Marlatt, G.A. *Assessment of addictive behaviors.* New York: Guilford, 1988.

This book unquestionably represents the state of the art on cognitive-behavioral assessment of substance-abuse problems. Of special interest are the chapters on the biopsychosocial model, assessment of expectancies regarding drinking, cannabis abuse, heroin addiction, and matching clients to treatment.

Donovan, J.M. An etiologic model of alcoholism. *American Journal of Psychiatry,* 1986, *143,* 1-11.

The author argues that failure to fully consider the multidimensional nature of the etiology of alcoholism has prevented research efforts from adequately integrating the contributions of heredity, environment, and psychopathology in a unified etiological model. He presents an outline of a multidimensional etiological model based on existing research findings.

Goodwin, D.W. Alcoholism and genetics: The sins of the fathers. *Archives of General Psychiatry,* 1985, *42,* 171-174.

This brief article is a good overview of what we can and cannot conclude about genetic influences in the etiology of alcoholism.

Hester, R., and Miller, W. *Handbook of alcoholism treatment approaches.* New York: Pergamon, 1989.

This book is of interest because it represents current thinking about cognitive-behavioral treatment of alcoholism. Some chapters we think especially thought provoking are those on "informed eclecticism," increasing motivation for change, antidipsotropic medications, self-control training (controlled drinking), and matching individuals with interventions.

Khantzian, E., Halliday, K., and McAuliffe, W. *Addiction and the vulnerable self: Modified dynamic group therapy for substance abusers.* New York: Guilford, 1990.

This solid book on group psychotherapy provides a practical guide to conducting a modified psychodynamically oriented group psychotherapy for cocaine addicts. It has application for other substance-abusing populations as well.

Khantzian, E.J. Psychotherapeutic interventions with substance abusers—The clinical context. *Journal of Substance Abuse Treatment,* 1985, *2,* 83-88.

Takes the position that ego deficits in the ability to tolerate painful affect and self-care capacities characterize many substance abusers. Suggests implications for treatment.

Kissin, B. Theory and practice in the treatment of alcoholism. In B. Kissin and H. Begleiter (Eds.), *The biology of alcoholism: (Vol. 5) Treatment and rehabilitation of the chronic alcoholic.* New York: Plenum, 1977, 1-48.

A classic, if somewhat overwhelming, overview of the biopsychosocial model of alcoholism.

Levy, M. A change in orientation: Therapeutic strategies for the treatment of alcoholism. *Psychotherapy,* 1987, *24(4),* 786-793.

Identifies several adjustments that psychodynamic therapists must make in order to work effectively with alcoholics: focus on the drinking itself, provide information about drinking problems and relapse prevention, maintain focus on the drinking as the treatment progresses, and carefully explore relapses.

Marlatt, G.A. Relapse prevention: Theoretical rationale and overview of the model In G. Marlatt and J. Gordon (Eds.), *Relapse prevention: Maintenance strategies in addictive behavior change.* New York: Guilford, 1985.

The first chapter in an impressive book presenting a cognitive-behavioral understanding of addiction and its treatment. The best single source on the relapse-prevention model.

Mendelson, J.H., and Mello, N.K. *The diagnosis and treatment of alcoholism.* New York: McGraw-Hill, 1985. (pp. 7, 10, 197-205, 221-231)

The indicated sections address the physiological and clinical features of alcohol dependence, and the variability of the syndrome, of the population, and of existing treatment methods.

Miller, W.R. Motivational interviewing with problem drinkers. *Behavioral Psychotherapy,* 1983, *11,* 147-172.

An important, provocative paper that defines "denial" as an interactional phenomenon and describes an approach to interviewing aimed at enhancing motivation for change.

Miller, W.R., and Hester, R.K. Inpatient alcoholism treatment: Who benefits? *American Psychologist,* 1986, *41,* 794-805.

Treatment outcome research is reviewed in order to compare the relative effectiveness of inpatient versus outpatient treatment.

Monti, P., Abrams, D., Kadden, R., and Cooney, N. *Treating alcohol dependence.* New York: Guilford, 1989.

A valuable resource for clinicians wishing to understand and to provide coping skills training. Included are a literature review and an explication of the theoretical rationale, as well as a wealth of practical, specific information on teaching communication, assertiveness, management of anger, and many other psychological and social skills.

Polich, J.M., Armor, D.J., and Braiker, H.B. Patterns of alcoholism over four years. *Journal of Studies on Alcohol,* 1980, *41,* 397-416.

This paper is based on the famous Rand Corporation follow-up study of alcoholics after treatment, which found the course of alcoholism to be variable across patients and suggested that more than one kind of remission might be possible. As such, it sparked controversy about whether controlled drinking might be a viable treatment goal.

Searles, J.S. The role of genetics in the pathogenesis of alcoholism. *Journal of Abnormal Psychology,* 1988, *97(2),* 153-167.

This careful critique of the research on the genetic basis of alcoholism by a researcher knowledgeable about behavior genetic methods is refreshingly thoughtful and objective at a time when biological factors are highly emphasized.

Sobell, L.C., Sobell, M.B., and Nirenberg, T.D. Behavioral assessment and treatment planning with alcohol and drug abusers: A review with an emphasis on clinical application. *Clinical Psychology Review*, 1988, *8*, 19-54.

Lists the types of information useful in a functional analysis of alcohol and drug use. Reviews a wide variety of assessment tools. Emphasizes a close relationship between assessment and treatment planning.

Steele, C., and Josephs, R. Alcohol myopia: Its prized and dangerous effects. *American Psychologist*, 1990, *45(8)*, 921-933.

Reports on programmatic research into the varied effect of alcohol on anxiety, depression, and social behavior. Using an information- processing paradigm, the authors and their colleagues compellingly explain diverse research findings.

Vannicelli, M. Group therapy with alcoholics: Special techniques. *Journal of Studies on Alcohol*, 1982, *43*, 17-37.

Identifies key issues and technical problems that arise in the interactional group treatment of substance abusers. Practical interventions are suggested that enable the clinician to respond effectively.

Vannicelli, M. Group therapy aftercare for alcoholic patients. *International Journal of Group Psychotherapy*, 1988, *38(3)*, 337-353.

This paper describes a dynamically oriented group aftercare program for alcoholics and other substance abusers pointing to the need for continuity of care, extending beyond the initial detoxification or initial crisis phase.

Vannicelli, M., Canning, D., and Griefen, M. Group therapy with alcoholics: A group case study. *International Journal of Group Psychotherapy*, 1984, *34*, 127-147.

Companion paper to the Vannicelli (1982) article, it presents detailed clinical examples of the techniques described by examining their use in a long-term group over the course of 2 years.

Washton, A. *Cocaine addiction: Treatment, recovery and relapse prevention.* New York: W. W. Norton, 1989.

An excellent text which is thoughtful, practical, and reflective of a state-of-the-art synthesis of treatment approaches and covers contracting, achieving abstinence, and relapse prevention. Although focused on cocaine addiction, it is very useful for thinking about treatment of alcohol and other drug abuse.

Weiss, R.D., and Mirin, S.M. Substance abuse as an attempt at self-medication. *Psychiatric Medicine*, 1987, *3*, 357-367.

Stresses the heterogeneity of the substance-abusing population and advises that several weeks of observation after the patient is drug- free may be needed to assess possible premorbid psychopathology.

Zucker, R.A. The four alcoholisms: A developmental account of the etiologic process. In C. Rivers (Ed.), *Alcohol and addictive behavior: Nebraska symposium on motivation, 1986.* Lincoln: University of Nebraska Press, 1987.

Offers a model for construing the influences on etiology of alcoholism as these influences vary over the course of individuals' development. Posits a set of types of alcoholism which differ in etiology.

Zucker, R.A., and Gomberg, E.S.L. Etiology of alcoholism reconsidered: The case for a biopsychosocial process. *American Psychologist,* 1986, *41,* 783-793.

Reviews longitudinal research on the etiology of alcoholism. Contrary to the increasingly prevalent view that alcoholism is predominantly a biological and genetic phenomenon, it concludes that childhood, personality, and cultural influences are important factors in the etiology of alcoholism.

Adult Children of Alcoholics

Bader, M.J. Looking for addictions in all the wrong places. *Tikkun,* 1988, *3(6), 13-16.*

A thoughtful article that examines important conceptual weaknesses and clinical pitfalls embedded in the ACOA self-help literature.

Brown, S. (1988). **Treating adult children of alcoholics: A developmental perspective.** New York: Wiley.

This book represents an important first step to systematically conceptualizing ACOA issues within a developmental model that makes use of family systems theory and developmental (primarily Piagetian) theory. The author stresses the importance of integrating a systems environmental view with theories of individual development.

Burk, J., and Sher, K. The "forgotten children" revisited: Neglected areas of COA research. *Clinical Psychology Review,* 1988, *8,* 285-302.

Aims to sensitize the reader to often-neglected considerations relevant to treatment of ACOAs, such as diversity of consequences of having an alcoholic parent, possible moderator variables affecting outcome, and the effects of labeling.

Hibbard, S. The diagnosis and treatment of adult children of alcoholics as a specialized therapeutic population. *Psychotherapy,* 1987, *24(4),* 779-785.

While recognizing the diversity of strengths and pathology among ACOAs, the author directs our attention to a set of frequently occurring pathogenic mechanisms in the life experience of the child with alcoholic parents.

Miller, R. 1987. Adult cousins of alcoholics. *Psychology of Addictive Behaviors, 1(1),* 74-76.

A humorous, satirical piece, that challenges the reader to think about the consequences of overlabeling.

Vannicelli, M. (1989). *Group psychotherapy with adult children of alcoholics: Treatment techniques and countertransference considerations.* New York: Guilford, 1989.

This book provides an overview of the ACOA literature, a rationale for group psychotherapy with the ACOA population, and focuses on special themes and issues that are likely to be salient in dynamically oriented psychotherapy groups with adult children of alcoholics. In addition, considerable emphasis is placed on countertransference issues and the leader's understanding of his own reactions as a vehicle for enhancing his work. Important myths and misconceptions in the ACOA literature are also challenged.

West, M., and Prinz, R. Parental alcoholism and childhood psychopathology. *Psychological Bulletin,* 1987, *102(2),* 204-218.

Reviews the literature on children of alcoholics published from 1975 to 1985. Underscores the variability in level of psychological functioning of COAs and summarizes the conclusions that can be drawn from existing research.

Wood, B.L. (1987). *Children of alcoholism: The struggle for self and intimacy in adult life.* New York: New York University Press.

This brief but well-written book examines ACOA issues from the perspective of object relations theory and self-psychology. Although the book addresses primarily the borderline ACOA, the author's crystal-clear exposition of self-psychology and object relations theory make this book a solid contribution to the ACOA literature.

Collaterals of Substance Abusers

Collins, R.L., Leonard, K.E., and Searles, J.S. *Alcohol and the family.* Guilford, 1990.

Although this is not a book that the reader will quickly zoom through (it is far too meaty), it offers an excellent resource for those embarking on research on any aspect of alcoholism and the family. It examines in depth the role of genetics in the development of alcoholism, the role of the family as a whole (its culture and dynamics), and the role of the marital dyad in developing and sustaining alcoholic behavior. In addition, parent-child processes and family dynamics that relate to the development of problem drinking in adolescence are explored.

Gaps between belief and knowledge are consistently highlighted, raising provocative questions for researchers as well as clinicians.

Gallant, D., and Mallott, D. Intervention techniques and married couples group therapy. In Zinberg, S., Wallace, J. and Bloom, S., (Eds.) *Practical approaches to alcoholism psychotherapy,* New York: Plenum, 1985.

A nice piece in terms of explicating—in brief format—what intervention is all about.

Johnson Institute. *How to use intervention in your professional practice.* Minneapolis: Johnson Institute Books, 1987.

An excellent small book. It offers the best practical guidance for facilitating an intervention by family and friends designed to make a substance-abusing loved one aware of the gravity of the problem and to motivate him to obtain treatment.

Kaufman, E. *Substance abuse and family therapy.* New York: Psychological Corporation (Harcourt, Brace, Jovanovich), 1985.

This is a highly readable classic integrating family systems and psychodynamic treatment approaches for working with substance-abusing families. The interplay between family dynamics and substance abuse is described in the section on family systems. The chapters on general principles of treatment with substance abusers, review of techniques, and the author's "personal synthesis" of treatment approaches are especially valuable.

Maxwell, R. *The booze battle,* New York: Ballantine Books, 1976.

This has a particularly good section on intervention that is useful for family members to read.

Steinglass, P., Bennett, L., Wolin, S., and Russ, D. *The alcoholic family.* New York: Basic Books, 1987.

Informed by family systems concepts, this exceptional piece of work describes programmatic research into the nature of the alcoholic family. Highly readable and clinically valuable.

Vannicelli, M. Treatment of alcoholic couples in outpatient group therapy. *Group,* 1987, *11(4),* 247-257.

This paper summarizes special issues that group leaders are likely to encounter when adapting their skills to outpatient group therapy with alcoholic couples, discussing the advantages of treating alcoholic couples in a group as opposed to individual couples therapy; the parameters of a couples group with alcoholic members that differentiate it from working with other kinds of couples in group; and techniques for tackling some of the specific kinds of problems and situations that arise.

❖ 12 ❖
Conclusion

We began this journey by looking backwards (Chapter 1) to a cultural context which had hindered effective delivery of services to substance abusers—a context in which substance abuse was regarded as a secondary problem and not given its due. As we conclude our journey, perhaps it is important to focus on the current context in which health care services are delivered to substance abusers and their family members and the challenges that lay ahead.

As this book is being written, the country is facing monumental changes in terms of delivery of health care services. Third-party payers (insurance companies) are increasingly reluctant to support lengthy inpatient hospital stays for psychiatric treatment and are escalating the criteria necessary to enter an inpatient facility—even for relatively brief periods of time. Gone are the days when a therapist's clinical opinion that it would be in the best interest of his patient to be hospitalized (along with some agreement on the part of his patient) would be sufficient to permit entry into an inpatient facility. And with inpatient psychiatric rates as high as $900.00 a day, even the very rich, without the help of third-party payers, are unable to make extensive use of in-hospital treatment.

Patients with substance-abuse problems have been among the hardest hit, with third-party payers even more reluctant to allow inpatient hospitalization for these individuals than for patients without substance-abuse diagnosis. This may, in part, be due to the fact that research investigators in the substance-abuse treatment field, examining the relative efficacy of inpatient versus outpatient treatment, have failed to demonstrate substantial advantages to inpatient treatment. The fact that the substance-abuse field has also developed a series of well-structured alternatives to inpatient treatment may also make it easier for third-party payers to hold back on inpatient care. Not only is the self-help network more fully developed in the substance-abuse field than in any other (it has, in fact, been a model for other mental health populations), but in addition, well-structured outpatient programs are available across the nation for treating substance abusers and their family members. Within the context of growing pressure to stem the tide of increasing health care costs, the inability of comprehensive outcome studies to document superior outcome for patients who are treated as inpatients over those treated as outpatients, combined with viable outpatient alternatives, understandably contributes to decreasing availability of inpatient services for substance abusers.

For mental health practitioners in the substance-abuse field, these changes offer a real challenge. With decreasing availability of inpatient services, outpatient services need to be more readily available at a cost that patients can afford. Fortunately, group psychotherapy makes this possible. The cost of group psychotherapy is roughly, hour-for-hour, one-third the cost of individual therapy; and outcome studies that have been done comparing group psychotherapy to individual therapy indicate that overall it is at least as effective. It is thus in the interest of our substance-abusing patients that the services of skilled clinicians be increasingly applied to delivering outpatient group psychotherapy services.

This book has attempted to provide the reader with a frame of reference for effectively providing group psychotherapy services to substance abusers and their family members. I have written as a clinician from my own personal experience—attempting to provide a map for future group leaders that will expedite their journey. Yet, to maximize the effective utilization of group psychotherapy, there is much territory that still needs to be systematically explored.

Clinical experience needs to be supplemented by research. More specifically, systematic studies are needed that will examine patient, leader, and group variables that are associated with positive outcome in group psychotherapy with these populations. For example, we need to know more about patient characteristics that facilitate "connecting" to a group. Because some patients are better able to connect to a group than others, it would also be instructive to know more about the particular characteristics that make this connection possible—that is, the personal characteristics that differentiate those patients who successfully engage (who continue membership, come regularly, and use the group productively) from those who do not. Thus, studies are needed that will focus on those particular personal attributes and strengths that enable a patient to use group therapy effectively, and on modifications in approach that may be useful for those patients who have more difficulty engaging. Although implicit in my writing is the assumption that most patients can substantially benefit from group psychotherapy—and that many will succeed far better in a group than in individual therapy—systematic data is needed to help us better understand which patients may have a harder time successfully utilizing the group and what changes in the basic parameters might make group therapy more useful for these patients (for example, more extensive preparation in the pregroup interviews, the use of individual therapy alongside of group therapy, and modifications in the structure of the group itself—length of sessions, activity level of the therapist, etc.).

Studies would also be of interest examining the limits of heterogeneity within a group; that is, how great a range—in level of functioning and other patient variables—can be effectively managed. In addition, studies might examine the relative efficacy for particular patient populations of therapy groups with different time frames—that is, of time-limited groups versus long-term groups without a time limit, compared to a third model in which patients come on board for a limited time period in which they contract to do a certain amount of work but have the option to renew membership within the framework of a long-term group.

Studies are also needed that will help us more crisply articulate the essential leader behaviors that help groups with these populations bond sufficiently to do the work of psychotherapy. Studies examining leader behavior within the first few sessions (activity level, norm-shaping behavior, and specific leader techniques to help patients to connect to one another) would be of interest, as would systematic investigation of many other aspects of the leader's behavior. In this book I have described a particular style of dynamically oriented group therapy and a particular therapeutic stance that characterizes the leader's behavior. Research would be helpful exploring the circumstances under which modification of this stance might be useful, and examining the efficacy of the stance that I have described (a relatively active, norm-shaping, nontransparent therapist) compared to a therapist stance that differs in some way from this.

Studies would also be useful examining the impact of the leader's past familial history with regard to substance abuse and the impact of this history on his effectiveness as a group leader. More specifically, this might include studies of frequency, intensity, and/or quality of countertransference reactions that may differentiate those group therapists who are recovering or who grew up in substance-abusing families from those without such a personal or familial history, and the particular troublespots that they may be more likely to encounter. Having more adequately investigated and systematically catalogued countertransference phenomena when working with substance abusers and their family members, we would then also be in a better position to explore the impact of countertransference training on leader skills and on clinical outcome with the populations described. Also useful would be studies that compare the impact of a single leader versus a co-leader team and the possible value of mixed teams in which one leader has a familial history related to substance abuse and the other one does not.

We also need to know more about the forces in the group itself that affect patient engagement and eventual outcome. Clinical experience tells us that there are some groups that more readily absorb new members and that seem to have a higher track record in terms of holding on to patients. More research is needed regarding the group culture —the group defensive maneuvers as well as the group adaptations that develop—that hinders or maximizes the "containing" elements of the group.

Studies are also needed regarding the effective ingredients for training the group therapist in the substance-abuse field. The balancing of substance-abuse knowledge with group-therapy knowledge (how much of each is needed) would be important to examine, as well as models for teaching and supervision. The apprenticeship model (in which a senior co-therapist works with a beginning therapist) might be compared to alternative models in which the beginning therapist proceeds on her own with close supervision via videotape or one-way mirror, or training models in which either of these two options is introduced only after the beginning therapist has observed groups (either as a recorder or behind a one-way mirror) for a period of time. Studies would also be useful examining various kinds of supervision for groups—for example, comparing group supervision in which a series of group therapists are supervised collectively and have an opportunity to hear about one another's groups, versus individual supervision of a single group at a time. Studies of the efficacy of countertransference supervision (which focuses heavily on what the group leader is experiencing as she conducts the group) versus supervision which focuses more specifically on the content of the patient's transactions would also be of interest.

In closing, I hope that the reader will carry away a sense of optimism and enthusiasm about conducting group psychotherapy with substance abusers and their family members, and a better sense of the territory involved as well as future directions. Toward this end I have provided guidelines for understanding the journey and for removing the roadblocks that are commonly encountered.

❖APPENDIX A❖
Population Estimates

POPULATION ESTIMATES OF LIFETIME AND CURRENT DRUG USE, 1988

The following are estimates of the number of people 12 years of age and older who report they have used drugs nonmedically. Drugs used under a physicians's care are not included. The estimates were developed from the 1988 National Household Survey on Drug Abuse and revised August 1989.

	12–17 yrs. (pop. 20,250,000)				18–25 yrs. (pop. 29,688,000)			
	%	Ever Used[b]	%	Current User[b]	%	Ever Used	%	Current User
Marijuana and hashish	17	3,516,000	6	1,296,000	56	16,741,000	16	4,594,000
Hallucinogens	3	704,000	1	168,000	14	4,093,000	2	569,000
Inhalants	9	1,774,000	2	410,000	12	3,707,000	2	514,000
Cocaine	3	683,000	1	225,000	20	5,858,000	5	1,323,000
Crack	1	188,000	*	*	3	1,000,000	1	249,000
Heroin	1	118,000	*	*	*	*	*	*
Stimulants	4	852,000	1	245,000	11	3,366,000	2	718,000
Sedatives	2	475,000	1	123,000	6	1,633,000	1	265,000
Tranquilizers	2	413,000	*	*	8	2,319,000	1	307,000
Analgesics	4	840,000	1	182,000	9	2,798,000	1	440,000
Alcohol	50	10,161,000	25	5,097,000	90	26,807,000	66	19,392,000
Cigarettes	42	8,564,000	12	2,389,000	75	22,251,000	35	10,447,000
Smokeless tobacco	15	3021,000	4	722,000	24	6,971,000	6	1,855,000

[a]Amounts of less than 0.5% are not listed and are indicated by asterisks.

[b]Terms: ever used; used at least once in a person's lifetime; current user; used at least once in th 30 days prior to the survey.

APPENDIX A *cont.*

		≥26 years (pop. 148,409,000)				TOTAL (pop. 198,347,000)		
%	Ever Used	%	Current User	%	Ever Used	%	Current User
31	45,491,000	4	5,727,000	33	65,748,000	6	11,616,000
7	9,810,000	*a	*	7	14,607,000	*	*
4	5,781,000	*	*	6	11,262,000	1	1,223,000
10	14,631,000	1	1,375,000	11	21,171,000	2	2,923,000
*	*	*	*	1	2,483,000	*	484,000
1	1,686,000	*	*	1	1,907,000	*	*
7	9,850,000	1	791,000	7	14,068,000	1	1,755,000
3	4,867,000	*	*	4	6,975,000	*	*
5	6,750,000	1	822,000	5	9,482,000	1	1,174,000
5	6,619,000	*	*	5	10,257,000	1	1,151,000
89	131,530,000	55	81,356,000	85	168,498,000	53	105,845,000
80	118,191,000	30	44,284,000	75	149,005,000	29	57,121,000
13	19,475,000	3	4,497,000	15	29,467,000	4	7,073,000

❖ *APPENDIX B* ❖
Appleton Outpatient
Clinic Diagram

Client Flow Through Appleton Outpatient Programs

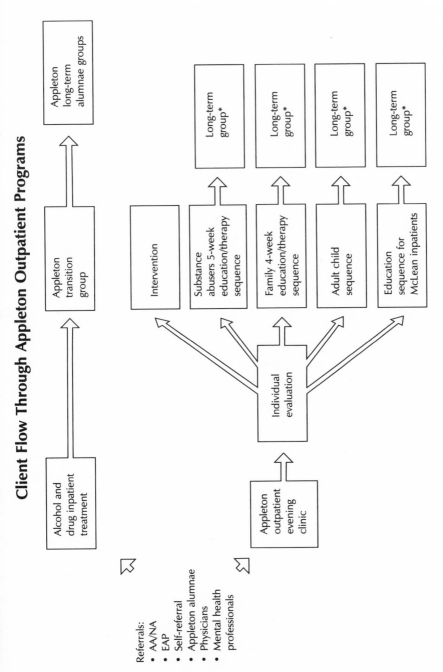

*Additional treatment modalities as indicated, including individual, couples, and family.

Referrals:
- AA/NA
- EAP
- Self-referral
- Appleton alumnae
- Physicians
- Mental health professionals

Alcohol and drug inpatient treatment

Appleton outpatient evening clinic

Individual evaluation

Intervention

Substance abusers 5-week education/therapy sequence

Family 4-week education/therapy sequence

Adult child sequence

Education sequence for McLean inpatients

Long-term group*

Long-term group*

Long-term group*

Long-term group*

Appleton transition group

Appleton long-term alumnae groups

❖ APPENDIX C ❖
Alcohol and Drug History Questionnaires

APPLETON DRUG/ALCOHOL DATA BASE

Name_____ Interviewer_____
    (Last)   (First)   (Middle)
                                                Date:_____

DEMOGRAPHIC DATA

Age_____ Marital Status_____
Race (circle)
    Father: Black   Caucasian   Asian   Other:_____
    Mother   Black   Caucasian   Asian   Other:_____
Ethnic group (circle)
    Father: Irish   French   English   Italian   Greek   Other:_____
    Mother: Irish   French   English   Italian   Greek   Other:_____
Religious Background (circle)
    Father: Protestant   Catholic   Jewish   Other   None
    Mother: Protestant   Catholic   Jewish   Other   None
    Patient: Protestant   Catholic   Jewish   Other   None
Education and Work History
    Patient's Education   # years_____ highest degree_____
    Father's Education   # years_____ highest degree_____
    Mother's Education   # years_____ highest degree_____
    Father's Occupation (descriptive title)
_____
    Mother's Occupation (descriptive title)
_____

Patient's Employment History:
    Best job (descriptive title)_____ when_____
    Occupation(s) in past year (descriptive titles)_____
_____

Number of jobs in past 3 years_____
Present employment status
    Paid: full-time_____; part-time_____ number of hours____
    Volunter: full-time_____; part-time_____ number of hours____
    Student: full-time_____; part-time_____ number of hours____
    Unemployed: Housewife/Mother_____ Retired_____ Other:_____
Day last worked_____
Total time in past 3 years out of work_____
If presently empoyed or a student:
    # days missed due to subtance abuse in month prior to treatment_____
    # days left early or arrived late due to substance abuse in month prior to
    treatment_____

RELATIVES' ALCOHOL/DRUG HISTORIES
Father

Has or has had alcohol/drug-abuse problem: yes_____ no_____
If yes: abuse ongoing_____ died from it_____ don't know_____
           recovering: number of months of total abstinence_____
           How? (AA/NA, therapy, Antabuse, etc.)_____
Drug(s) of choice: alcohol_____ cocaine_____ cannabis_____ opiate_____
           minor tranquilizer_____ other_____
Drinking: alcoholic_____ heavy_____ moderate_____ little_____ none_____

Mother

Has or has had alcohol/drug-abuse problem: yes_____ no_____
If yes: abuse ongoing_____ died from it_____ don't know_____
           recovering: number of months of total abstinence_____
           How? (AA/NA, therapy, Antabuse, etc.)_____
Drug(s) of choice: alcohol_____ cocaine_____ cannabis_____ opiate_____
           minor tranquilizer_____ other_____
Drinking: alcoholic_____ heavy_____ moderate_____ little_____ none_____

Other relatives with substance-abuse problems

(sibling, step-parent, aunt/uncle, grandparent, fiance, former spouse)

Nature of relationship_____
Recovering_____ abuse ongoing_____ died from it_____ don't know_____
Drug(s) of choice: alcohol_____ cocaine_____ cannabis_____ opiate_____
           minor tranquilizer_____ other_____

Nature of relationship_____
Recovering_____ abuse ongoing_____ died from it_____ don't know_____
Drug(s) of choice: alcohol_____ cocaine_____ cannabis_____ opiate_____
           minor tranquilizer_____ other_____

Nature of relationship_____
Recovering_____ abuse ongoing_____ died from it_____ don't know_____
Drug(s) of choice: alcohol_____ cocaine_____ cannabis_____ opiate_____
           minor tranquilizer_____ other_____

Nature of relationship_____
Recovering_____ abuse ongoing_____ died from it_____ don't know_____
Drug(s) of choice: alcohol_____ cocaine_____ cannabis_____ opiate_____
           minor tranquilizer_____ other_____

RECENT ALCOHOL/DRUG HISTORY

When was last drink/drug use?_____
Why stopped alcohol/drug use?_____

Identifiable precipitant of most recent increase in patient's level of alcohol/drug use?
yes_____ no_____ no increase_____
If yes, describe:_____

Intensity of current preoccupations with using alcohol or drugs:
High____ moderate____ minimal____

MOTIVATION FOR CURRENT TREATMENT

Check degree of motivation for each category at left:

	Great	Moderate	Little
Family pressure			
Employer pressure or job loss			
Concern about physical health			
Legal pressure			
Therapist pressure			
Personal distress			
Overall motivation			

SUBSTANCE-ABUSE HISTORY

Age of first drink_____   Age of onset of heavy drinking_____
Age of first drug use_____   Age of onset of heavy drug use_____

Identifiable precipitant of onset of alcohol/drug abuse? yes____ no____
If yes, describe:_____

Longest period totally alcohol- and drug-free since heavy use began_____
Longest period abstinent from drug of choice since heavy use began_____

Alcohol/drug use during heaviest one month period of abuse (age=____):

	Average days/week	Quantity/day
Alchohol		
Cocaine		
Cannabis		
Other:_____		
Other:_____		
Other:_____		

Include minor tranquilizers, opiates, etc. (even if prescribed).
Use specific names of "other" drugs.
For *Quantity*: give representative range, specify IV use, freebase.

Alcohol/drug use during most recent period of abuse:
(check if same as above_____)

	Average days/week	Quantity/day
Alchohol		
Cocaine		
Cannabis		
Other:_____		
Other:_____		
Other:_____		

Predominat pattern of drinking/drug use: Binge____ Maintenance____

Social patters of drinking/drug use (most recent period of abuse):
alone____ with others____ home____ work____ social settings____

PATTERNS OF CHANGE IN USAGE

Since the age that alcohol and/or drugs became problematic, at what ages did you notice marked *changes* in use; and what patterns do you recognize that relate to these changes? (ask patient to draw a timeline and graph if this will help)

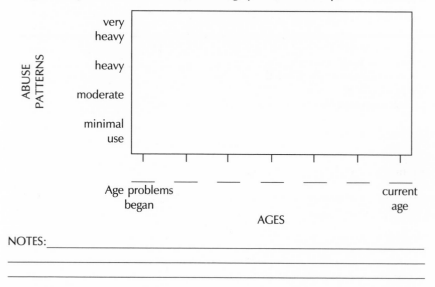

NOTES:_____

_____

_____

_____

SYMPTOMS

Alcohol-related symptoms:

	Age first noticed	Number of occurrences in past year
Blackouts.................		
Memory deficit.............		
Tremors (shakes)...........		
Hallucinations.............		
Numbness.................		
Uncoordination............		
Blurred vision.............		
Other:_____		

Check if no alcohol-related symptoms_____

Drug-related symptoms:

	Age first noticed	Number of occurrences in past year
Tremors (shakes)...........		
Profuse sweating...........		
Nausea..................		

	Age first noticed	Number of occurrences in past year
Vomiting..................		
Dry heaves................		
Poor appetite..............		
Weight loss................		
Diarrhea..................		
Seeing things not there......		
Hearing voices.............		
Feeling things under skin.....		
Seizures; convulsions........		
Insomnia..................		
Heart attack/stroke..........		
Other:_____		

Check if no drug-related symptoms_____

LEGAL PROBLEMS

Number of arrests *directly related to drinking or durg use* (e.g., DWI, drunk and disorderly, possession, dealing): past year_____ total_____
    Specific types of charges:_____

Number of *other* arrests: year_____ total_____
    Specific types of charges:_____

Illicit method used to obtain or pay for drugs: dealing_____ theft_____
    prostitution_____ other:_____ none_____

Current legal problems (court actions pending, divorce suits, custody suits, DWI, litigation, etc.):_____
_____

SOCIAL/INTERPERSONAL COMPLICATIONS OF SUBSTANCE USE

The extent to which substance use has been asociated with:
    (1) breaking one's own standard with regard to sexual conduct (poorer choice in partner, greater number, etc.)_____
                                        (considerable, some, minimal)
    (2) health risks (AIDS-risk behaviors such as needle sharing, failure to practice safe sex) _____
                                (considerable, some, minimal)

PROBLEMS WITH LEISURE TIME

Extent to which drinking and drugging currently substitute for productive leisure time activities: considerably_____ some_____ minimally_____

Availability of hobbies and interests: never had any_____
    In past enjoyed:_____
    Currently enjoy:_____

PREVIOUS TREATMENT

Outpatient treatment for substance abuse:

	Number of times used				Age ranges when treatment occurred
	None	1–5	6–20	21+	
Substance-abuse counseling .					
Group therapy					
Antabus					
AA/NA					
Other:_____					
Other:_____					

If AA/NA minimally used in past, does this relate to spirituality concerns and issues, problem with higher power, etc.? yes_____ no_____

Inpatient treatment for substance abuse:
    Total number of hospitalizations_____ Duration of longest_____
    Age ranges when treatment occured_____

Other outpatient treatment:

	Number of times used				Age ranges when treatment occurred
	None	1–5	6–20	21+	
Individual therapy					
Group therapy					
Couple/family therapy					
Other:_____					
Other:_____					

    Major tranquilizers ever? yes_____ no_____ If yes, age_____
    Antidepressants ever? yes_____ no_____ If yes, age_____

Other inpatient treatment:
    Total number of hospitalizations_____ Duration of longest_____
    Age ranges when treatment occured_____

APPLETON ACOA DATA BASE

Name_____ Interviewer_____
    (Last)   (First)   (Middle)
                                        Date:_____

RELATIVES' ALCOHOL/DRUG HISTORIES

Father

Has or has had alcohol/drug-abuse problem: yes_____ no_____
If yes: abuse ongoing_____ died from it_____ don't know_____
          recovering: number of months of total abstinence_____
          How? (AA/NA, therapy, Antabuse, etc.)_____
Drug(s) of choice: alcohol_____ cocaine_____ cannabis_____ opiate_____
                minor tranquilizer____ other_____
Drinking: alcoholic_____ heavy_____ moderate_____ little_____ none_____

Mother

Has or has had alcohol/drug-abuse problem: yes_____ no_____
If yes: abuse ongoing_____ died from it_____ don't know_____
          recovering: number of months of total abstinence_____
          How? (AA/NA, therapy, Antabuse, etc.)_____
Drug(s) of choice: alcohol_____ cocaine_____ cannabis_____ opiate_____
                minor tranquilizer____ other_____
Drinking: alcoholic_____ heavy_____ moderate_____ little_____ none_____

Other relatives with subtance-abuse problems

(sibling, step-parent, aunt/uncle, grandparent, fiance, former spouse)

Nature of relationship_____
Recovering_____ abuse ongoing_____ died from it____ don't know____
Drug(s) of choice: alcohol____ cocaine_____ cannabis_____ opiate_____
                minor tranquilizer____ other_____

Nature of relationship_____
Recovering_____ abuse ongoing_____ died from it____ don't know____
Drug(s) of choice: alcohol____ cocaine_____ cannabis_____ opiate_____
                minor tranquilizer____ other_____

Nature of relationship_____
Recovering_____ abuse ongoing_____ died from it____ don't know____
Drug(s) of choice: alcohol____ cocaine_____ cannabis_____ opiate_____
                minor tranquilizer____ other_____

Nature of relationship_____
Recovering_____ abuse ongoing_____ died from it____ don't know____
Drug(s) of choice: alcohol_____ cocaine_____ cannabis_____ opiate_____
                   minor tranquilizer____ other_____
Nature of relationship_____
Recovering_____ abuse ongoing_____ died from it____ don't know____
Drug(s) of choice: alcohol_____ cocaine_____ cannabis_____ opiate_____
                   minor tranquilizer____ other_____

RECENT ALCOHOL/DRUG HISTORY

When was last drink/drug use?_____
If no longer using, why stopped alcohol/drug use?_____
_____

If recent increase in use, was there an identifiable precipitant? yes____ no____
no sudden increase____ If yes, describe:_____
_____

Alcohol/drug use during past year:

	Average days/week	Quantity/day
Alcohol.		
Cocaine		
Cannabis.		
Other:_____		
Other:_____		
Other:_____		

Predominant pattern of drinking/drug use: Light social_____
Heavy social_____ Binge_____ Maintenance_____

Social context of drinking/drug use (past year):
alone_____ with others_____ home_____ work_____ social settings_____

Used alcohol with other CNS depressants (e.g., Valium, opiates): yes_____ no_____
If presently empoyed or a student:
days missed due to subtance abuse in month prior to treatment_____
days left early or arrived late due to substance abuse in month prior to
treatment_____
days in past 3 years missed work or school because of substance use_____

PAST SUBSTANCE USE HISTORY

Age of first drink_____   Age of onset of heaviest drinking_____
Age of first drug use_____   Age of onset of heaviest drug use_____

Identifiable precipitant of changes in pattern (or onset of alchohol/drug use)?
yes____ no____ If yes, describe:_____

Longest alcohol- and drug-free period in heaviest drinking/drug use years_____
Longest drug-of-choice-free period in heaviest drinking/drug use years_____

Alcohol/drug use during heaviest one month period (age=_____):

	Average days/week	Quantity/day
Alchohol		
Cocaine		
Cannabis		
Other:_____		
Other:_____		
Other:_____		

Include minor tranquilizers, opiates, etc, (even if prescribed).
Use specific names of 'other' drugs.
For *Quantity*: give representative range, specify IV use, freebase.

SYMPTOMS

Alcohol-related symptoms:

	Age first noticed	Number of occurrences in past year
Blackouts		
Memory deficit.		
Tremors (shakes).		
Hallucinations.		
Numbness.		
Uncoordination		
Blurred vision		
Other:_____		
Other:_____		

Check if no alcohol-related symptoms_____

Drug-related symptoms:

	Age first noticed	Number of occurrences in past year
Temors (shakes)		
Profuse sweating		
Nausea		
Vomiting.		
Dry heaves		
Poor appetite		
Weight loss.		
Diarrhea		
Seeing things not there		
Hearing voices		
Feeling things under skin		

	Age first noticed	Number of occurrences in past year
Seizures; convulsions		
Insomnia		
Other:_____		
Other:_____		

Check if no drug-related symptoms_____

LEGAL PROBLEMS

Number of arrest *directly related to drinking or durg use* (e.g., DWI, drunk and disorderly, possession, dealing): past year_____ total_____
  Specific types of charges:_____

Number of *other* arrests: year_____ total_____
  Specific types of charges:_____

Illicit method used to obtain or pay for drugs: dealing_____ theft_____
  prostitution_____ other:_____ none_____

PREVIOUS TREATMENT
Substance Abuse Treatment
Outpatient Treatment

	Number of times used				Age ranges when treatment occurred
	None	1–5	6–20	21+	
Substance-abuse counseling .					
Group therapy					
Antabus					
Naltrexone					
AA/NA					
Other:_____					
Other:_____					

Inpatient treatment

  Total number of hospitalizations_____ Duration of longest_____
  Age ranges when treatment occurred_____

Other Psychiatric Treatment
Outpatient treatment:

	Number of times used				Age ranges when treatment occurred
	None	1–5	6–20	21+	
Individual therapy					
Group therapy					
Couple/family therapy					

	Number of times used				Age ranges when
	None	1–5	6–20	21+	treatment occurred
Behavioral therapy					
Other:_____					
Other:_____					

Major tranquilizers ever? yes_____ no_____ If yes, age_____
Antidepressants ever? yes_____ no_____ If yes, age_____

Inpatient treatment:

Total number of hospitalizations_____ Duration of longest_____
Age ranges when treatment occurred_____

❖ APPENDIX D ❖
Michigan Alcoholism Screening Test and Scoring Key

PATIENT:_____

DATE:_____

EVALUATOR_____

QUESTIONNAIRE ABOUT DRINKING PROBLEMS

Directions: If a statement says something true about you, put a check (✓) in the nearby space under YES. If a statement says something not true about you, put a check in the nearby space under NO. Please answer all the questions.

	YES	NO
1. Do you feel you are a normal drinker?	____	____
2. Have you ever awakened the morning after some drinking the night before and found that you could not remember a part of that evening?	____	____
3. Does your spouse (or parents) ever worry or complain about your drinking?	____	____
4. Can you stop drinking without a struggle after one or two drinks?	____	____
5. Do you ever feel bad about your drinking?	____	____
6. Do friends or relatives think you are a normal drinker?	____	____
7. Do you ever try to limit your drinking to certain times of the day or to certain places?	____	____
8. Are you always able to stop drinking when you want to?	____	____
9. Have you ever attended a meeting of Alcoholics Anonymous (AA)?	____	____
10. Have you gotten into fights when drinking?	____	____
11. Has drinking ever created problems with you and your spouse?	____	____
12. Has your spouse (or other family member) ever gone to anyone for help about your drinking?	____	____
13. Have you ever lost friends or girlfriends or boyfriends because of your drinking?	____	____
14. Have you ever gotten into trouble at work because of your drinking?	____	____
15. Have you ever lost a job because of your drinking?	____	____
16. Have you ever neglected your obligations, your family or your work for two or more days in a row because you were drinking?	____	____
17. Do you ever drink before noon?	____	____

18. Have you ever been told you have liver trouble? ____ ____

19. Have you ever had delirium tremens (DTs), severe ____ ____
shaking, heard voices or seen things that weren't there
after heavy drinking?

20. Have you ever gone to anyone for help about your ____ ____
drinking?

21. Have you ever been in a hospital because of your ____ ____
drinking?

22. Have you ever been a patient in a psychiatric hospital or ____ ____
on a psychiatric ward of a general hospital where
drinking was part of the problem?

23. Have you ever been seen in a psychiatric or mental ____ ____
health clinic, or gone to a doctor, social worker, or
clergyman for help with an emotional problem in which
drinking played a part?

24. Have you ever been arrested, even for a few hours, ____ ____
because of drunk behavior?

25. Have you ever been arrested for drunk driving or driving ____ ____
after drinking?

SCORING KEY TO MAST

Directions for scoring: Add together point values for all items on which points are earned, to classify patient as: *social drinker* (total score of 0–2 points); *borderline* (total score of 3–4 points); or *alcoholic* (total score of 5 and above).

	YES	NO
1. Do you feel you are a normal drinker?		2
2. Have you ever awakened the morning after some drinking the night before and found that you could not remember a part of that evening?	2	
3. Does your spouse (or parents) ever worry or complain about your drinking?	1	
4. Can you stop drinking without a struggle after one or two drinks?		2
5. Do you ever feel bad about your drinking?	1	
6. Do friends or relatives think you are a normal drinker?		2
7. Do you ever try to limit your drinking to certain times of the day or to certain places?		
8. Are you always able to stop drinking when you want to?		2
9. Have you ever attended a meeting of Alcoholics Anonymous (AA)?	5*	
10. Have you gotten into fights when drinking?	1	
11. Has drinking ever created problems with you and your spouse?	2	
12. Has your spouse (or other family member) ever gone to anyone for help about your drinking?	2	
13. Have you ever lost friends or girlfriends or boyfriends because of your drinking?	2	
14. Have you ever gotten into trouble at work because of your drinking?	2	
15. Have you ever lost a job because of your drinking?	2	
16. Have you ever neglected your obligations, your family or your work for two or more days in a row because you were drinking?	2	

---

*Discretion may be indicated in scoring this item to account for those who accompanied an alcoholic family member to a meeting.

17. Do you ever drink before noon?   1   _____

18. Have you ever been told you have liver trouble?   2   _____

19. Have you ever had delirium tremens (DTs), severe   5   _____
    shaking, heard voices or seen things that weren't there
    after heavy drinking?

20. Have you ever gone to anyone for help about your   5   _____
    drinking?

21. Have you ever been in a hospital because of your   5   _____
    drinking?

22. Have you ever been a patient in a psychiatric hospital or   2   _____
    on a psychiatric ward of a general hospital where
    drinking was part of the problem?

23. Have you ever been seen in a psychiatric or mental   2   _____
    health clinic, or gone to a doctor, social worker, or
    clergyman for help with an emotional problem in which
    drinking played a part?

24. Have you ever been arrested, even for a few hours,   2   _____
    because of drunk behavior?

25. Have you ever been arrested for drunk driving or driving   2   _____
    after drinking?

❖ APPENDIX E ❖
Group Ground Rules

APPLETON OUTPATIENT PSYCHOTHERAPY GROUP GROUND RULES

The behavior and feelings of members of the therapy group mirror in important ways behavior and feelings in other important relationships. Consequently, the group provides a setting in which to examine patterns of behavior in relationships. The group also provides a context in which members learn to identify, understand and express their feelings. The therapist's role is to facilitate this group process.

To foster these goals, we believe that several group ground rules are important. These are as follows:

1. Members joining long-term groups remain as long as they find the group useful in working on important issues in their lives. We recommend at least a year. Members are required to make an initial 3-month commitment in order to determine the usefulness of this particular group for them.

2. Regular and timely attendance at all sessions is expected. As a member, it is your responsibility to notify the group in advance when you know that you will be away or late for group. In the event of and unexpected absence, you should notify the group at least 24 hours in advance to avoid being charged for the missed session.

3. Members of Appleton substance-abuse groups are committed to maintaining abstinence. If a relapse does occur, it must be discussed promptly in the group—as must thoughts or concerns about resuming drug/alcohol use. Members of ACOA and family groups are asked to be reflective about their own susbstance use and to bring up changes in patterns of use or concerns that mey be associated with use.

4. Members will notify the group if they are considering leaving the group. Because leaving the group is a process, just as joining is, members are expected to see this process through for at least 3 weeks following notification of termination.

5. Members will have a commitment to talk about important issues in their lives that cause difficulty in relating to others or in living life fully.

6. Members will also have a commitment to talk about what is going on in the group itself as a way of better understanding their own interpersonal dynamics.

7. Members will treat matters that occur in the group with utmost confidentiality. To that end, members are expected not to discuss what happens in the group with people who are not members of the group.

8. Outside-of-group contact often has considerable impact on the group's therapeutic effectiveness. Therefore, any relevant interactions between members which occur outside the group should be brought back into the next meeting and shared with the entire group.

9. What you share in the group will be shared with other members of the treatment team when we feel that it is important to your treatment to do so.

10. Payments for group are due at the last meeting of the month unless other arrangements are discussed and explicitly worked out in the group. If for any reason timely payment becomes problematic, members are expected to discuss this in the group.

❖APPENDIX F❖
Dimensions of the Therapeutic Contract

GROUND RULES TO CONSIDER

EXPECTATIONS FOR PATIENT

1. *Fees*
   a. Amount of fee
   b. Fee increases (frequency and amount)
   c. Fee reductions (basis for decision and criteria for re-evaluation)
   d. Payment schedule (weekly, monthly)
   e. Payment format (mailed in response to bill, paid at beginning of session, paid at end of session)
   f. Policy regarding owing money
   g. Amount of advance notice to avoid paying for canceled sessions
   h. How insurance forms will be handled

2. *Frequency of sessions*
   a. Number of session per week
   b. Scheduling additional time when needed
   c. Policy regarding sessions that fall on Holidays

3. *Between-session contacts*
   a. Scheduling extra time
   b. Availability for telephone contact
      (1) Length of calls and frequency that will be permitted
      (2) Whether calls will be charged or not
      (3) Hours that are permissible (anytime day or night? weekends?)
   c. Outside contact (and socializing) among group members

4. *Length of sessions*
   a. Usual length
   b. Session length if patient comes late

5. *Regularity of attendance and promptness* (especially important for group)

6. *Initial evaluation* (specifying number of sessions to decide if therapist and the patient will work together)

7. *Length of treatment*

8. *Expectations regarding what and how patient will share*
   a. How silences will be dealt with
   b. Whether patient is told he is there to talk about whatever comes to mind and that he will provide the agenda

9. *Talking about, rather than acting on, feelings*
   a. Physical contact
   b. Threatening or destructively abusive verbal behavior

10. *Confidentiality* (especially important for group)

11. *Planning termination* (especially important for group)

EXPECTATIONS FOR THERAPIST

1. *Reliability* (keeping appointments)
2. *Promptness* (on time for appointments)
   a. How therapist will handle sessions that he comes late for (will time be made up?)
3. *Therapist's self-disclosure*
   a. Topics that are acceptable
   b. Topics that are not acceptable
   c. Whether this will be addressed at the outset or will come up topic by topic
4. *Physical contact*
   a. Handshakes
   b. Hand on shoulder
   c. Other
5. *Giving advice*
   a. About what topics
   b. When this is considered appropriate
6. *Rescheduling appointments*
   a. Based on patient's needs
   b. Based on therapist's needs
7. *Returning phone meassages* (how soon?)
8. *Confidentiality* (with whom the therapist will discuss the case and release-of-information forms)
9. *Keeping awake and alert during sessions*

❖APPENDIX G❖
Clinical Face Sheet

CLINICAL FACE SHEET

I. PATIENT DEMOGRAPHICS

Patient Name:_____

Date of Birth:_____ Ins. Co. and #:_____

Contact Person in Case of Emergency:_____

Home Address:_____

Telephone: Home:_____ Work:_____

II. TREATMENT CONTRACT

Fee:

    Amount:_____

    Scheduling of Payments:_____

    Billing Party (Direclty to Patient or to Insurance Company):_____

    Schedule for Review of Rates or Increases in Fee:_____

Length of Session:_____

Cancellation Policy:_____

_____

III. CONTACT WITH OTHER TREATERS:

Therapist 1: Name_____

             Phone:_____

             Permission to Contact: Yes/No

Therapist 2: Name_____

             Phone:_____

             Permission to Contact: Yes/No

❖ References ❖

Ackerman, R.J. (Ed.). (1986). *Growing in the shadow.* Pompano Beach, FL: Health Communications.

Ackerman, R.J. (1987). *Same house different homes.* Pompano Beach, FL: Health Communications.

Alexander, F. (1948). *Fundamentals of psychoanalysis.* New York: W.W. Norton.

Alexander, J., & Alexander, R. (1991). *Recovery plus: Freedom from co-dependency.*Deerfield Beach, FL: Health Communications.

Alonso, A. (1987). Discussion of "Women's groups led by women." *International Journal of Group Psychotherapy, 37*(2), 159.

Alpert, G. (1988). *Rapid turnover groups: Therapist techniques for facilitating the development of productive group process.* Unpublished manuscript.

American Psychiatric Association. (1987). *Diagnostic and statistical manual of mental disorders* (3rd ed., rev.). Washington, DC: American Psychiatric Association.

Bader, M.J. (1988). Looking for addictions in all the wrong places. *Tikkun 3*(6), 13–16.

Beattie, M. (1987). *Co-dependent no more: How to stop controlling others and start caring for yourself.* New York: Harper/Hazelden.

Beattie, M. (1990a). *Co-dependents guide to the twelve steps.* New York: Prentice Hall.

Beattie, M. (1990b). *The language of letting go: Daily meditations for co-dependents.* New York: Harper & Row.

Becnel, B.C. (1989). *Parents who help their children overcome drugs.* Minneapolis, MN: CompCare.

Beletsis, S.G., & Brown, S. (1981). A developmental framework for understanding the adult children of alcoholics. *Journal of Addictions and Health, 2*(4), 187–203.

Berry, R.E., Jr., Boland, J.P., Smart, C.N., & Kanak, J.R. (1977). *The economic costs of alcohol abuse and alcoholism—1975 (Final Report to National Institute of Alcohol Abuse and Alcoholism under Contract No. ADM 281–76–0016).* Boston: Policy Analysis. Bion, W.R. (1961). *Experiences in groups.* New York: Basic Books.

Bion, W.R. (1962). *Learning from experience.* New York: Basic Books.

Birke, S. & Mayer, K. (1990). *Together we heal: A real life portrait of recovery in group therapy for adult children.* New York: Ballantine.

Black, C. (1981). *It will never happen to me!* Denver: M.A.C. Publications.

Black, C. (1985). *Repeat after me.* Denver: M.A.C. Publications.

Blane, H.T., & Leonard, K.E. (Eds.). (1987). *Psychological theories of drinking and alcoholism*. New York: Guilford.

Blume, S.B. (1985). Group psychotherapy in the treatment of alcoholism. In S. Zimberg, J. Wallace, & S.Blume (Eds.), *Practical approaches to alcoholism psychotherapy (2nd edition)*. New York: Plenum.

Bohman, M., Sigvardsson, S., & Cloninger, C.R. (1981). Maternal inheritance of alcohol abuse. *Archives of General Psychiatry, 38*(9), 965–969.

Bolman, L. (1971). Some effects of trainers on their T groups. Journal of Applied Behavioral Science, 7(3), 309–325.

Bolman, L. (1973). Some effects of trainers on their groups: A partial replication. *Journal of Applied Behavioral Science, 9*(4), 534–539.

Brandsma, J.M., & Pattison, E.M. (1985). The outcome of group psychotherapy alcoholics: An empirical review. *American Journal of Drug and Alcohol Abuse, 11*(1 & 2), 151–160.

Brix, D.J. (1983). Use of a group-centered psychotherapy group with the inpatient treatment of alcoholism, *Bulletin of the Society of Psychologists in Addictive Behaviors, 2*(4), 253–258.

Brown, S. (1988). *Treating adult children of alcoholics: A developmental perspective.* New York: Wiley.

Brown, S., & Beletsis, S. (1986). The development of family transference in groups for the adult children of alcoholics. *International Journal of Group Psychotherapy, 36*(1), 97–114.

Brown, S., & Yalom, I.D. (1977). Interactional group therapy with alcoholics. *Journal of Studies on Alcohol, 38*(3), 426–456.

Brownell, K.D., Marlatt, G.A., Lichtenstein, E., & Wilson, G.T. (1986). Understanding and preventing relapse. *American Psychologist, 41*(7), 765–782.

Brunner-Orne, M. (1956). The utilization of group psychotherapy in enforced treatment programs for alcoholics and addicts. *International Journal of Group Psychotherapy 6*, 272–279.

Burk, J.P., & Sher, K.J. (1988). The "forgotten children" revisited: Neglected areas of COA research. *Clinical Psychology Review, 8*, 285–302.

Cadogan, D.A. (1973). Marital group therapy in the treatment of alcoholism. *Quarterly Journal of Studies on Alcohol, 34*(4), 1187–1194.

Cahalan, D. (1976). *Problem drinkers: A national survey*. San Francisco: Jossey-Bass.

Carnes, P. (1989). *A gentle path through the twelve steps: A guidebook for all people in the process of recovery*. Minneapolis, MN: CompCare.

Cermak, T.L. (1985). *A primer on adult children of alcoholics*. Pompano Beach, FL: Health Communications.

Cermak, T.L., & Brown, S. (1982). Interactional group therapy with the adult children of alcoholics. *International Journal of Group Psychotherapy, 32*(3), 375–389.

Clark, W.B., & Cahalan, D. (1976). Changes in problem drinking over a four-year span. *Addictive Behaviors, 1*, 251–259.

Clark, W.B., & Midanik, L. (1982). Alcohol use and alcohol problems among U.S. adults. In *Alcoholic consumption and related problems (Alcohol and Health Monograph no.1)*. Rockville, MD: NIAAA.

Cloninger, C.R. (1987). Neurogenetic adaptive mechanisms in alcoholism. *Science,* 236, 410–416.

Collet, L. (1990). After the anger, what then. *The Family Therapy Networker, 14*(1), 22–31.

Collins, R.L., Leonard, K.E., & Searles, J. S. (Eds.). (1990). *Alcohol and the family: Research and clinical perspectives.* New York: Guilford.

Cook, D.R. (1985). Craftsman versus professional: Analysis of the controlled drinking controversy. *Journal of Studies on Alcohol, 46*(5), 433–442.

Cooper, D.E. (1987). The role of group psychotherapy in the treatment of substance abusers. *American Journal of Psychotherapy, 41*(1), 55–67.

Cooper, D.E. (1988). *Role requirements of the group psychotherapist: Empathy and neutrality.* Paper presented at the annual meeting of the American Group Psychotherapy Association, New York.

Corder, B.S., Corder, R.S., & Laidlaw, N.P. (1972). An intensive program for alcoholics and their wives. *Quarterly Journal of Studies on Alcohol, 33,* 1144–1146.

Corder, B.F., McRee, C., & Rohrer, H. (1984). *Daughters of alcoholics: A review of the literature.* North Carolina Journal of Mental Health, 10(20), 37–43.

Corey, M., & Corey, G. (1987). *Group: Process and practice* (3rd ed.) Monterey, CA: Brooks/Cole.

Davis, D.I., Berenson, D., Steinglass, P., & Davis, S. (1974). The adaptive consequences of drinking. *Psychiatry, 37,* 209–215.

Dick, B., Lessler, K., & Whiteside, J. (1980). A developmental framework for cotherapy. *International Journal of Group Psychotherapy, 30*(3), 273–283.

Dies, R.R. (1983). Clinical implications of research on leadership in short-term group psychotherapy. In R.R. Dies & K.R. Mackenzie (Eds.), *Advances in group psychotherapy: Integrating reasearch and practice.* New York: International Universities Press.

Dies, R.R., & Cohen, L. (1976). Content considerations in group therapist self-disclosure. *International Journal of Group Psychotherapy, 26*(1), 71–88.

Dies, R.R., Mallet, J., & Johnson, F. (1979). Openness in the coleader relationship: Its effect on group process and outcome. *Small Group Behavior, 10*(4), 523–546.

Donovan, D.M., & Marlatt, G.A. (1980). Assessment of expectancies and behaviors associated with alcohol consumption. *Journal of Studies on Alcohol, 41*(11), 1153–1185.

Donovan, D.M., & Marlatt, G.A. (1988). *Assessment of addictive behaviors.* New York: Guilford.

Donovan, J.M. (1986). An etiologic model of alcoholism. *American Journal of Psychiatry, 143*(1), 1–11.

Doroff, D.R. (1977). Group psychotherapy and alcoholism. In B. Kissin & H. Begleiter (Eds.), *The biology of alcoholism: Vol. 5, Treatment and rehabilitation of the chronic alcoholic.* ew York: Plenum.

Drews, T.R. (1980). *Getting them sober: A guide for those living with alcoholism.* Plainfield, NJ: Bridge.

Ebersole, G.O., Leiderman, P.H., & Yalom, I.D. (1969). Training the non-professional group therapist: A controlled study. *The Journal of Nervous and Mental Diseases, 149*(3), 294–302.

Elder, I.R. (1990). *Conducting group therapy with addicts: A guidebook for professionals.* Blue Ridge Summit: Tab Books.

Emrick, C. (1975). A review of psychologically oriented treatment of alcoholism II: The relative effectiveness of different treatment approaches and the effectiveness of treatment vs. no treatment. *Journal of Studies on Alcohol, 36*(1), 88–108.

Epstein, L. (1979). The therapeutic use of countertransference data with borderline patients. *Contemporary Psychoanalysis, 15*(2), 248–275.

Fairbairn, W.R.D. (1981). The repression and the return of bad objects. In *Psychoanalytic studies of the personality* (7th ed.). London: Routledge & Kegan Paul. (Original work published in 1943)

Forrest, G.G. (1986). *How to live with a problem drinker and survive.* New York: Macmillan.

Fox, R. (1962). Group psychotherapy with alcoholics. *International Journal of Group Psychotherapy, 12*(1), 56–63.

Frank, D.J. (1985). Therapeutic components shared by all psychotherapies. In M. Mahoney & A. Freeman (Eds.), *Cognition and Psychotherapy.* New York: Plenum.

Friedman, W.H. (1989). *Practical group therapy: A guide for clinicians.* San Francisco: Jossey-Bass.

Friel, J.C., & Friel, L.D. (1988). *Adult children: The secrets of dysfunctional families.* Deerfield Beach, FL: Health Communications.

Gallant, D., & Mallott, D.M. (1985). Intervention techniques and married couples group therapy. In S. Zinberg, J. Wallace, and S. Bloom, (Eds.), *Practical approaches to alcoholism psychotherapy.* New York: Plenum Press.

Gallup, G., & Newport, F. (1990). Americans now drinking less alcohol. *The Gallup Poll News Service, 55*(31), 1–3.

Goodwin, D.W. (1985). Alcoholism and genetics: The sins of the fathers. *Archives of General Psychiatry, 42,* 171–174.

Goodwin, D.W., Schulsinger, F., Hermansen, L., Guze, S.B., & Winokur, G. (1973). Alcohol problems in adoptees raised apart from alcoholic biological parents. *Archives of General Psychiatry, 28,* 238–243.

Gordis, E. (Ed.). (1987). *Alcohol and health: Sixth special report to the Congress (U.S. Department of Health and Human Services, publication No. ADM 87–1519).* Washington, DC: US Government Printing Office.

Gravitz, H.L., & Bowden, J.D. (1984). Therapeutic issues of adult children of alcoholics. *Alcohol Health and Research World, 8*(4), 25–36.

Gravitz, H.L., & Bowden, J.D. (1985). *Guide to recovery: A book for adult children of alcoholics.* Holmes Beach, FL: Learning Publications.

Greenleaf, J. (1981). *Co-alcoholic, para-alcoholic: Who's who and what's the difference?* Denver: M.A.C. Publications.

Griefen, M., Vannicelli, M., & Canning, D. (1985). Treatment contracts in long-term groups with alcoholic outpatients: A group case study. *Group, 9*(3), 43–48.

Grotstein, J. (1981). *Splitting and projective identification.* New York: Jason Aronson.

Guntrip, H. (1969). *Schizoid phenomena, object relations and the self* (7th ed.). New York: International Universities Press.

Hedlund, J.L., & Vieweg, B.W. (1984). The Michigan Alcoholism Screening Test (MAST): A comprehensive review. *Journal of Operational Psychiatry, 15,* 55–65.

Heilfron, M. (1969). Co-therapy: The relationship between therapists. *International Journal of Group Psychotherapy, 19*(3), 366–381.

Hester, R., & Miller, W. (Eds.). (1989). *Handbook of alcoholism treatment approaches: Effective alternatives.* New York: Pergamon.

Hibbard, S. (1987). The diagnosis and treatment of adult children of alcoholics as a specialized therapeutic population. *Psychotherapy, 24*(4), 779–785.

Hindman, M.H. (1979). Family violence. *Alcohol Health and Research World, 4*(1), 1–11

Holder, H.D. (1987). Alcoholism treatment and potential health care cost saving. *Med Care, 25*(1), 52–71.

Honig, F., & Spinner, A. (1986). A group therapy approach in the treatment of spouses of alcoholics. *Alcoholism Treatment Quarterly, 3*(3), 91–105.

Hurley, J.R., & Force, E.J. (1973), T-group gains in acceptance of self and others. *International Journal of Group Psychotherapy, 23*(2), 166–176.

Igersheimer, W. (1959). Group psychotherapy for the non-alcoholic wives of alcoholics. *Quarterly Journal of Studies on Alcohol, 20,* 77–85.

Imhof, J., Hirsch, R., & Terenzi, R.E. (1983). Countertransferential and attitudinal considerations in the treatment of drug abuse and addiction. *The International Journal of the Addictions, 18*(4), 491–510.

Jellinek, E.M. (1960). *The disease concept of alcoholism.* New Haven, CT: College and University Press.

Johnson, V.E. (1986). *Intervention: How to help someone who doesn't want help.* Minneapolis: Johnson Institute Books.

Johnson Institute. (1987). *How to use intervention in your professional practice.* Minneapolis: Johnson Institute Books.

Kanas, N. (1982). Alcoholism and group psychotherapy. In E.M. Pattison & E. Kaufman (Eds.), *Encyclopedic handbook of alcoholism* (pp. 1011–1021). New York: Gardner Press.

Kanfer, F.H., & Schefft, B.K. (1988). *Guiding the process of therapeutic change.* Champaign, IL: Research Press.

Kaufman, E. (1985). *Substance abuse and family therapy.* New York: The Psychological Corporation/Harcourt Brace Jovanovich.

Khantzian, E.J. (1985). Psychotherapeutic interventions with substance abusers—The clinical context. *Journal of Substance Abuse Treatment, 2,* 83–88.

Khantzian, E.J., Halliday, K.S., & McAuliffe, W.E. (1990). *Addiction and the vulnerable self: Modified dynamic group therapy for substance abusers.* New York: Guilford.

Kissin, B. (1977). Theory and practice in the treatment of alcoholism. In B. Kissin & H. Begleiter (Eds.), *The biology of alcoholism: Vol. 5, Treatment and rehabilitation of the chronic alchoholic.* New York: Plenum.

Kozel, N.J., & Adams, E.H. (Eds.). (1985). Cocaine use in America: Epiodemiologic and clinical perspectives. *NIDA Research Monographs, 61.*

Kritsberg, W. (1985). *The adult children of alcoholics syndrome: From discovery to recovery.* Pompano Beach, FL: Health Communications.

Langs, R.J. (1975). The therapeutic relationship and deviations in technique. *International Journal of Psychoanalytic Psychotherapy, 4,* 106–141.

Levin, J.D. (1987). *Treatment of alcoholism and other addictions: A self-psychology approach.* Northvale, NJ: Jason Aronson.

Levine, R. (1988). Contributions of countertransference data from the analysis of the Rorschach: An object-relations approach. In H.D. Lerner & P.M. Lerner (Eds.), *Primitive mental states and the Rorschach.* Madison, CT: International Universities Press.

Levy, M. (1987). A change in orientation: Therapeutic strategies for the treatment of alcoholism. *Psychotherapy, 24*(4), 786–793.

Lieberman, M.A. (1983). Comparative analysis of change mechanisms in groups. In R.R. Dies & K.R. MacKenzie (Eds.), *Advances in group psychotherapy: Integrating research and practice.* New York: International University Press.

Lieberman, M.A., Yalom, I.D., & Miles, M.B. (1973). *Encounter groups: First facts.* New York: Basic Books.

Malin, A., & Grotstein, J.S. (1966). Projective identification in the therapeutic process. *The International Journal of Psycho-Analysis, 47*(1), 26–31.

Marlatt, G.A. (1985). Relapse prevention: Theoretical rationale and overview of the model. In G. Marlatt & J. Gordon (Eds.), *Relapse prevention: Maintenance, strategies in the treatment of addictive behaviors.* New York: Guilford.

Maxwell, R. (1976). *The booze battle.* New York: Ballantine Books.

McCarthy, R.G. (1946). Group therapy in an outpatient clinic for the treatment of alcoholism. *Quarterly Journal of Studies on Alcohol, 7,* 98–109.

McCarthy, R.G. (1949). Group therapy in alcoholism. Transcription of a series of sessions recorded in an outpatient clinic. I. Introduction and first two sessions. *Quarterly Journal of Studies on Alcohol, 10,* 63–108.

McConnell, P. (1980). *Adult children of alcoholics: A workbook for healing.* San Francisco: Harper & Row.

McConnell, P. (1986). *A workbook for healing: Adult children of alcoholics.* New York: Harper & Row.

McCrady, B.S., Moreau, J., Paolino, T.J., Jr., & Longabaugh, R. (1982). Joint hospitalization and couples therapy for alcoholism; A four-year follow-up. *Journal of Studies on Alcohol, 43*(11), 1244–1250.

McCrady, B.S., Noel, N.E., Abrams, D.B., Stout, R.L., Nelson, H.F., & Hay, W.M. (1986). Comparative effectiveness of three types of spouse involvement in outpatient behavioral alcoholism treatment. *Journal of Studies on Alcohol, 47*(6), 459–467.

McCrady, B.S., Paolino, T.J., Jr., Longabaugh, R., & Rossi, J. (1979). Effects of joint hospital admission and couples treatment for hospitalized alcoholics: A pilot study. *Addictive Behaviors, 4*(2), 155–165.

McDonnell, R., & Callahan, R. (1987). *Hope for healing: Good news for adult children of alcoholics.* New York: Paulist Press.

Mellody, P., & Miller, A.W. (1989). *Breaking free: A recovery workbook for facing co-dependence.* New York: Harper & Row.

Mendelson, J.H., & Mello, N.K. (Eds.). (1985). *The diagnosis and treatment of alcoholism (2nd ed.).* New York: McGraw-Hill.

Middelton-Moz, J., & Dwinell, L. (1986). *After the tears: Reclaiming the personal losses of childhood.* Pompano Beach, FL: Health Communications.

Miller, W.R. (1983). Motivational interviewing with problem drinkers. *Behavioural Psychotherapy, 11*, 147–172.

Miller, W.R. (1987). *Adult cousins of alcoholics. Psychology of Addictive Behaviors, 1*(1), 74–76.

Miller, W.R., & Hester, R.K. (1986). Inpatient alcoholism treatment: Who benefits? *American Psychologist, 41*(7), 794–805.

Miller, J.E., & Ripper, M.L. (1988). *Following the yellow brick road: The adult child's personal journey through Oz*. Deerfield Beach, FL: Health Communications.

Monti, P.M., Abrams, D.B., Kadden, R.M., & Cooney, N.L. (1989). *Treating alcohol dependence*. New York: Guilford.

Moos, R.H., & Billings, A.G. (1982). Children of alcoholics during the recovery process: Alcoholic and matched control families. *Addictive Behaviors, 7*, 155–163.

Moos, R.H., Finney, J.W., & Chan, D.A. (1981). The process of recovery from alcoholism: I. Comparing alcoholic patients and matched community controls. *Journal of Studies on Alcohol, 42*(5), 393–402.

Moos, R.H., & Moos, B.S. (1984). The process of recovery from alcoholism: III. Comparing functioning in families of alcoholics and matched control families. *Journal of Studies on Alcohol, 45*(2), 111–118.

Mueller, L.A., & Ketcham, K. (1987). *Recovery: How to get and stay sober*. New York: Bantam Books.

Mummey, J. (1987). *The joy of being sober: A book for recovering alcoholics and those who love them*. Chicago: Contemporary Books.

National Institute on Drug Abuse. (1989). Population estimates of lifetime and current drug use, 1988. Washington, DC: NIDA.

Nuckols, C.C. (1989). *Cocaine: From dependency to recovery* (2nd ed.). Bradenton, FL: Human Services Institute.

O'Connel, K.R. (1985). *End of the line: Quitting cocaine*. Philadelphia: Westminster Press.

O'Farrell, T.J., Cutter, H.S., & Floyd, F.J. (1985). Evaluating behavioral marital therapy for male alcoholics: Effects on marital adjustment and communication from before to after treatment. *Behavior Therapy, 16*(2), 147–169.

Paine-Gernee, K., & Hunt, T. (1990). *Emotional healing: A guide to overcoming the wounds of the past and building a healthy future*. New York: Warner Books.

Paolino, T.J., Jr., & McCrady, B.S. (1976). Joint admission as a treatment modality for problem drinkers: A case report. *American Journal of Psychiatry, 133*(2), 222–224.

Pattison, E.M. (1985). The selection of treatment modalities for the alcoholic patient. In J.H. Mendelson & N.K. Mello (Eds.), *The diagnosis and treatment of alcoholism* (2nd ed.). New York: McGraw-Hill.

Perez, J.F. (1986). *Counseling the alcoholic group*. New York: Gardner Press.

Pittman, B. (1988). *Stepping stones to recovery*. Seattle, WA: Glen Abbey Books.

Polich, J.M., Armor, D.J., & Braiker, H.B. (1980). Patterns of alcoholism over four years. *Journal of Studies on Alcohol, 41*(5), 397–416.

Polich, J.M., Armor, D.J., & Braiker, H.B. (1981). *The course of alcoholism four years after treatment*. New York: Wiley.

Porterfield, K.M. (1984). *Keeping promises: The challenge of a sober parent.* San Francisco: Harper & Row.

Racker, H. (1968). *Transference and countertransference.* Madison, CT: International Universities Press.

Roberts, M.C.F., Floyd, F.J., O'Farrell, T., & Cutter, H.S.G. (1985). Marital interactions and the duration of alcoholic's husbands' sobriety. *American Journal of Drug and Alcohol Abuse, 11,* 303–313.

Robins, L.N., Helzer, J.E., Weissman, M.M., Orvaschel, H., Gruenberg, E., Burke, J.D., & Regier, D.A. (1984). Lifetime prevalence of specific psychiatric disorders in three sights. *Archives of General Psychiatry, 41*(10), 949–958.

Russell, M., Henderson, C., & Blume, S.B. (1985). *Children of alcoholics: A review of the literature.* New York: Children of Alcoholics Foundation.

Rutan, J.S., Alonso, A., & Molin, R. (1984). Handling the absence of group leaders: To meet or not to meet. *International Journal of Group Psychotherapy, 34*(2), 273–287.

Rutan, J.S., & Stone, W.N. (1984). *Psychodynamic group psychotherapy.* New York: Macmillan.

Sands, P.M., & Hanson, P.G. (1971). Psychotherapeutic groups for alcoholics and relatives in an outpatient setting. *International Journal of Group Psychotherapy, 21*(1), 23–33.

Saxe, L., Dougherty, D., Esty, J., & Fine, M. (1983). *The effectiveness and costs of alcoholism treatment (Congressional Office of Technology Assessment Case Study, Publication No. 052–003–00902–1).* Washington, DC: US Government Printing Office.

Schlesinger, S.E., & Horberg, L.K. (1988). *Taking charge: How families can climb out of addiction and flourish.* New York: Simon & Schuster.

Schuckit, M.A., Li, T.K., Cloninger, C.R., & Deitrich, R.A. (1985). Genetics of alcoholism. *Alcoholism: Clinical and Experimental Research, 9*(6), 475–492.

Schuckit, M.A., & Morrisey, E.R. (1976). Alcoholism in women: Some clinical and social perspectives with an emphasis on possible subtypes. In M. Greenblatt & M.A. Schuckit (Eds.), *Alcoholism problems in women and children.* New York: Grune & Stratton.

Scida, J., & Vannicelli, M. (1979). Sex-role conflict and women's drinking. *Journal of Studies on Alcohol, 40*(1), 28–44.

Scott, E.M. (1955). A special type of group therapy and its application to alcoholics. *Quarterly Journal of Studies on Alcohol, 17*(2), 288–290.

Searles, H.F. (1979). *Countertransference and related subjects.* New York: International Universities Press.

Searles, J.S. (1988). The role of genetics in the pathogenesis of alcoholism. *Journal of Abnormal Psychology, 97*(2), 153–167.

Secil, C. (1990). *Wisdom to recover by: Study topics for people growing up in sobriety.* Minneapolis: CompCare.

Seixas, J.S., & Levitan, M.L. (1984). A supportive counseling group for adult children of alcoholics. *Alcoholism Treatment Quarterly, 1*(4), 123–132.

Seixas, J.S., & Youcha, G. (1985). *Children of alcoholism: A survivor's manual.* New York: Harper & Row.

Selzer, M.L. (1971). The Michigan Alcoholism Screening Test: The quest for a new diagnostic instrument. *American Journal of Psychiatry, 127*(12), 1653–1658.

Selzer, M.L., Vinokur, A., & van Rooijen, L. (1975). A self-administered Short Michigan Alcoholism Screening Test (SMAST). *Journal of Studies on Alcohol, 36*(1), 117–126.

Shaffer, H.J., & Gambino, B. (1990). Epilogue: Integrating treatment choices. In H.B. Milkman & L.I. Sederer (Eds.), *Treatment choices for alcoholism and substance abuse.* Lexington, MA: Lexington Books.

Smith, A.W. (1988). *Grandchildren of alcoholics: Another generation of co-dependency.* Deerfield Beach, FL: Health Communications.

Smith, C.C. (1990). *Recovery at work: A clean and sober career guide.* San Francisco: Harper/Hazelden.

Sobell, M.B., & Sobell, L.C. (1973a). Individualized behavior therapy for alcoholics, *Behavior Therapy, 4*(1), 49–72.

Sobell, M.B., & Sobell, L.C. (1973b). Alcoholics treated by individualized behavior therapy: One year treatment outcome. *Behaviour Research and Therapy, 11,*599–618.

Sobell, M.B., & Sobell, L.C. (1976). Second year treatment outcome of alcoholics treated by individualized behavior therapy: Results. *Behaviour Research and Therapy, 14*(3), 195–215.

Sobell, L.C., Sobell, M.B., & Nirenberg, T.D. (1988). Behavioral assessment and treatment planning with alcohol and drug abusers: A review with an emphasis on clinical application. *Clinical Psychology Review, 8,*19–54.

Solomon, S.D. (1983). Individual versus group therapy: Current status in the treatment of alcoholism. *Advances in Alcohol and Substance Abuse, 2*(1), pp. 69–86.

Steele, C. M., & Josephs, R. A. (1990). Alcohol myopia: Its prized and dangerous effects. *American Psychologist, 45*(8), 921–933.

Steiner, C.M. (1977). *Games alcoholics play.* New York: Grove Press.

Steinglass, P. (1979a). The alcoholic family in the interaction laboratory. *Journal of Nervous and Mental Disease, 167*(7), 428–436.

Steinglass, P. (1979b). An experimental treatment program for alcoholic couples. *Journal of Studies on Alcohol, 40*(3), 159–182.

Steinglass, P., Bennett, L.A., Wolin, S.J., & Reiss, D. (1987). *The alcoholic family.* New York: Basic Books.

Steinglass, P., Davis, D.I., & Berenson, D. (1977). Observations of conjointly hospitalized "alcoholic couples" during sobriety and intoxication: Implications for theory and therapy. *Family Process, 16,* 1–16.

Subby, R. (1990). Healing the family within. Deerfield Beach, FL: Health Communications.

Vaillant, G.E. (1983). *The natural history of alcoholism: Causes, patterns, and paths to recovery.* Cambridge, MA: Harvard University Press.

Vaillant, G.E., Clark, W., Cyrus, C., Milofsky, E.S., Kopp, J., Wulsin, V.W., & Mogielnicki, N.P. (1983). Prospective study of alcoholism treatment: Eight-year follow-up. *American Journal of Medicine, 75,* 455–463.

Vannicelli, M. (1978). *Impact of aftercare in the treatment of alcoholics: A cross-lagged panel analysis, 39*(11), 1875–1886.

Vannicelli, M. (1982). Group psychotherapy with alcoholics: Special techniques. *Journal of Studies on Alcohol, 43*(1), 17–37.

Vannicelli, M. (1987). Treatment of alcoholic couples in outpatient group therapy. *Group, 11*(4), 247–257.

Vannicelli, M. (1988). Group therapy aftercare for alcoholic patients. *International Journal of Group Psychotherapy, 38*(3), 337–353.

Vannicelli, M. (1989). *Group psychotherapy with adult children of alcoholics:·Treatment techniques and countertransference considerations.* New York: Guilford.

Vannicelli, M. (1991). Dilemmas and countertransference consideration in group psychotherapy with adult children of alcoholics. *International Journal of Group Psychotherapy, 41*(3), pp. 295–312.

Vannicelli, M. (1990). Group psychotherapy with adult children of alcoholics. In M. Seligman & L.A. Marshall (Eds.), *Group psychotherapy: A practitioner's guide to interventions with special populations.* Boston: Allyn & Baron.

Vannicelli, M., Canning, D., & Griefen, M. (1984). Group therapy with alcoholics: A group case study. *International Journal of Group Psychotherapy, 34*(1), 127–147.

Vannicelli, M., Dillavou, D., & Caplan, C. (1988). *Dynamically oriented group therapy with alcoholics: Making it work despite the prevailing bias.* Paper presented at American Group Psychotherapy Association Meeting, New York.

Vannicelli, M., Gingerich, S., & Ryback, R. (1983). Family problems related to the treatment and outcome of alcoholic patients. *British Journal of Addiction, 78,*193–204.

Vinogradov, S., & Yalom, I.D. (1989). *A concise guide to group psychotherapy.* Washington: American Psychiatric Press.

Washton, A.M. (1989). *Cocaine addiction: Treatment, recovery, and relapse prevention.* New York: W.W. Norton.

Washton, A.M., Gold, M.S., & Pottash, A.C. (1986). *Treatment outcome in cocaine abusers. In L.S. Harris (Ed.), Problems of drug dependence 1985: Proceedings of the 47th Annual Scientific Meeting, The Committee of Drug Dependence.* NIDA Research Monograph 67. Rockville, MD: NIDA.

Wegscheider-Cruse, S. (1985). *Choice-making for co-dependents, adult children and spirituality seekers.* Pompano Beach, FL: Health Communications.

Weigel, R.G., Dinges, N., Dyer, R., & Straumfjord, A.A. (1972). Perceived self-disclosure, mental health, and who is liked in group treatment. *Journal of Counselling Psychology, 19,* 47–52.

Weisman, M.N., & Robe, L.B. (1983). *Relapse/slips: Abstinent alcoholics who return to drinking.* Minneapolis: Johnson Institute.

Weiss, R.D., & Mirin, S.M. (1987). Substance abuse as an attempt at self-medication. *Psychiatric Medicine, 3,* 357–367.

West, M., & Livesley, W.J. (1986). Therapist transparency and the frame for the group. *International Journal of Group Psychotherapy, 36*(3), 5–19.

West, M.O., & Prinz, R.J. (1987). Parental alcoholism and childhood psychopathology. *Psychological Bulletin, 102*(2), 204–218.

Whitfield, C.I. (1987). *Healing the child within: Discovery and recovery for adult children of dysfunctional families.* Deerfield Beach, FL: Health Communications.

Winnicott, D.W. (1949). Hate in the countertransference. *The International Journal of Psycho-Analysis, 30*(2), 69–74.

Winnicott, D.W. (1965). *The maturational processes and the facilitating environment.* New York: International Universities Press.

Winnicott, D.W. (1975). Clinical varieties of transference. In D.W. Winnicott (Ed.). *Through paediatrics to psycho-analysis.* New York: Basic Books. (Original work published in 1955)

Winokur, G. (1974). The division of depressive illness into depressive spectrum disease and pure depressive disease. *International Pharmacopsychiatry, 9*(1), 5–13.

Winokur, G. (1979). Alcoholism and depression in the same family. In D.W.G. Goodwin and C.K. Erickson (Eds.), *Alcoholism and affective disorders: Clinical genetic and biochemical studies.* New York: SP Medical and Scientific Books.

Wiseman, J.P. (1981). Sober comportment, patterns and perspectives on alcohol addiction. *Journal of Studies on Alcohol, 42,* 106–126.

Woititz, J.G. (1983). *Adult children of alcoholics.* Pompano Beach, FL: Health Communications.

Woititz, J.G. (1985). *Struggle for intimacy.* Pompano Beach, FL: Health Communications.

Wolberg, L.R. (1948). *Medical hypnosis* (Vol. 1). New York: Grune & Stratton.

Wolin, S.J., Bennett, L.A., & Noonan, D.L. (1979). Family rituals and the recurrence of alcoholism over generations. *American Journal of Psychiatry, 136*(4B), 589–593.

Wood, B.L. (1987). *Children of alcoholism: The struggle for self and intimacy in adult life.* New York: New York University Press.

Woodruff, R.A., Guze, S.B., Clayton, P.J., and Carr, D. (1973). Alcoholism and depression. *Archives of General Psychiatry, 28,* 97–100.

Wright, K.D., & Scott, T.B. (1978). The relationship of wives' treatment to the drinking status of alcoholics. *Journal of Studies on Alcohol, 39,* 1577–1581.

Yalom, I.D. (1970). *The theory and practice of group psychotherapy.* New York: Basic Books.

Yalom, I.D. (1974). Group therapy and alcoholism. *Annals of the New York Academy of Sciences, 233,* 85–103.

Yalom, I.D. (1975). *The theory and practice of group psychotherapy* (2d ed.). New York: Basic Books.

Yalom, I.D. (1990). *Love's executioner.* New York: Basic Books.

Zimberg, S. (1982). Psychotherapy in the treatment of alcoholism. In E.M. Pattison & E. Kaufman (Eds.), *Encyclopedic handbook of alcoholism.* New York: Gardner.

Zucker, R.A. (1987). The four alcoholisms. A developmental account of the etiologic process. In C. Rivers (Ed.), *Alcohol and addictive behavior: Nebraska Symposium on Motivation, 1986.* Lincoln: University of Nebraska Press.

Zucker, R.A., & Gomberg, E.S.L. (1986). Etiology of alcoholism reconsidered: The case for a biopsychosocial process. *American Psychologist, 41*(7), 783–793.

❖Index❖

DATE DUE